Hispanic Aged Mental Health

Hispanic Aged Mental Health

T. L. Brink, PhD
Editor

The Haworth Press, Inc.
New York • London • Norwood (Australia)

Hispanic Aged Mental Health has also been published as *Clinical Gerontologist*, Volume 11, Numbers 3/4 1992.

The Haworth Press, Inc. 10 Alice Street, Binghamton, NY 13904-1580 USA

Library of Congress Cataloging-in-Publication Data

Hispanic aged mental health / T.L. Brink, editor.
   p. cm.
   Has also been published as Clinical gerontologist, volume 11, numbers 3/4, 1992.
   Includes bibliographical references and index.
   ISBN 1-56024-107-1 (H : alk. paper). – ISBN 1-56024-217-5 (S : alk. paper)
   1. Hispanic American aged – Mental health. 2. Hispanic American aged – Mental health services. I. Brink, T. L. (Terry L.)
   [DNLM: 1. Hispanic Americans. 2. Mental Health – in old age. 3. Mental Health Ser-
vices – in old age. W1 CL71D v. 11 no. 3/4]
RC451.5.H57H57 1992
618.97′689′008968073 – dc20
DNLM/DLC
for Library of Congress
                                                92-1473
                                                  CIP

Hispanic Aged Mental Health

Hispanic Aged Mental Health

CONTENTS

SECTION THREE: ASSESSMENT OF SPECIAL
  PROBLEMS

SECTION FOUR: SERVICE UTILIZATION

ABOUT THE EDITOR

T. L. Brink, PhD, is currently on the faculty of Crafton Hills College in Yucalpa, California, and Iberoamerican University in Mexico City, Mexico. He is a member of the International Council of Psychologists, the International Psychogeriatric Association, the National Social Science Association, and the Western Psychological Association. The American Psychological Association named him a Distinguished Visitor in 1984.

During his career, Dr. Brink has developed the International Version of the Mental Status Questionnaire, the Geriatric Depression Scale, the Hypochondriasis Scale (Institutional Geriatric), the Scale for Paranoia (Observer Rated Geriatric), and the Stimulus Recognition Test. His books include *Geriatric Psychotherapy* (Human Sciences Press, 1969; Imago, 1983); *The Middle Class Credo* (R&E, 1984; Fawcett Gold Medal, 1985); *Clinical Gerontology: A Guide to Assessment and Intervention* (The Haworth Press, Inc., 1986); *The Elderly Uncooperative Patient* (The Haworth Press, Inc., 1987); and *Mental Health in the Nursing Home* (The Haworth Press, Inc., 1990). He has published over 250 articles, chapters and reviews. Dr. Brink has been the editor of the journal *Clinical Gerontologist* since 1982.

Introduction

This book began as a special issue of *Clinical Gerontologist: The Journal of Aging and Mental Health*. Societal, cross-cultural, and ethnic factors had been the topic in various full-length articles, clinical comments and reviews in previous issues of CG:

1984 III (1) 79-80
1984 III (2) 40-41
1985 IV (1) 51-52
1986 IV (3) 56-58
1986 IV (4) 29-35, 66-68, 74-75
1988 VIII (2) 63-83, 115-116, 120
1989 VIII (4) 72-73
1990 X (1) 79
1990 X (2) 109

The editor lives in Mexico, a Mexican psychiatrist is on our editorial board, and previous issues have contained several articles written by physicians, psychologists, social workers and nurses from Mexico and Argentina, as well as Spanish Speaking mental health professionals in the U.S., yet few articles dealt specifically with the mental health of Hispanic aged. Ironically, the only full-length article devoted specifically to Hispanic aged was in the premier issue of Clinical Gerontologist:

1982 I (1) 51-58

Since that time, books written in Spanish, or translated into Spanish, have been reviewed in the journal, but only one book specifically on Latin American mental health:

1985 IV (1) 92

and none on Latin American or Hispanic aged.

It was therefore decided to put together this special issue and book, and emphasize a clinically-relevant presentation of mental health issues in this population. Dozens of submissions were received on this topic, and se-

1

lecting the final contributors to this volume was difficult. The following chapters differ greatly in terms of length, level of theoretical speculation, and breadth of coverage of previous research. What unites them is their relevance to practitioners dealing with mental health issues in the Hispanic aged.

It is hoped that this volume will open up more work with this population. The editor hopes that in the future more articles, clinical comments and reviews can be published on the Hispanic aged.

TLB

SECTION ONE:
SUCCESSFUL AGING

Chapter One

Diversity of Aging Experience in Latin America and the Caribbean

Luis Alberto Vargas, MD, PhD

Editor's Introduction

Vargas begins this volume by shattering the fallacious image of the generic (and hence, stereotypical) Hispanic. Diversity describes the different Hispanic culture(s) on this continent. Variables such as population growth and migration, as well as differences in history, political systems, and economic development, account for the diversity.

LATIN AMERICA AND THE CARIBBEAN

The American continent is varied from both a natural and a sociocultural perspective. The people that lived in it before the Old World and the New World met, ranged from tribes of hunters and gatherers with a Paleo-

Luis Alberto Vargas is an MD and he holds a PhD in Biological Anthropology. The author works as a full time researcher at the Instituto de Investigaciones Antropológicas of the National University of Mexico. He is a member of the Mexican National Academy of Medicine, and president of the Mexican Association of Biological Anthropology. He has been a visiting professor in several American universities, and was a consultant for a year and a half at the Pan American Health Organization in Washington DC, where he obtained most of the information for this article.

Dr. Vargas wishes to thank Dr. Elías Anzola, Regional Advisor on the Program on health for the Elderly of PAHO for his support, and access to materials cited in this article.

Address correspondence and requests for reprints to: Dr. Luis Alberto Vargas, Ingeneiros 55, Miguel Hidalgo, D.F., 11800 Mexico.

5

lithic technology to nations that had achieved knowledge and technology that in some aspects was more advanced than the ones of their conquerors. After 1492, South of the United States, the ways of the Old and New Worlds amalgamated and gave birth to a new and different way of life.

From a social and cultural perspective, the countries of the Americas can be classified the following way:

1. *North America*, encompassing Canada and the United States of America.
2. *The Caribbean*, which can be subdivided in:
   a. The English speaking countries.
   b. The Spanish speaking countries and territories (Cuba, the Dominican Republic and Puerto Rico).
   c. Haiti.
   d. The European territories and colonies.
3. *Latin America* geographically is part of North, Central and South America, and includes all the countries South of the United States of America in which Spanish or Portuguese is spoken. Although Cuba and the Dominican Republic are in the Caribbean, culturally they are akin to the Latin American countries. From a cultural perspective, these countries can be divided in those with:
   a. A large Indian population and a cosmopolitan minority (for example: Perú, Bolivia, Guatemala).
   b. A small or nonexistent Indian population and a cosmopolitan majority (for example: Costa Rica, Argentina).
   c. The *mestizo* countries, where Indians, Negroes, Europeans and others have intermarried, although some ethnic minorities may remain (for example: México, Brazil, Nicaragua).

Mestizo is the Spanish word for hybrid, that is the offspring of living beings of different biological stock. But *mestizo* is also used in a larger sense, to include culture. Many of the Latin American societies are truly a mixture of the Iberian culture (including its Jewish and Arabic components) with that of the Indians that lived before the arrival of the Europeans, the slaves brought from Africa, and all the later immigrants. This is reflected in their way of life: despite the powerful influence of the United States, France, England, Japan and other countries, Latin America maintains its identity, based on the use of the Spanish and the Portuguese languages, and reinforced through a common heritage of music, literature and other arts. Latin Americans do have a sense of being *Latinos*.

MAJOR DEMOGRAPHIC AND SOCIOECONOMIC CHANGES IN THE AREA

This century, Latin America has suffered a series of changes that affect the situation of the elderly. Among the most important of them are:

Population Increase

Latin America and the Caribbean are two of the areas in the world with the greatest demographic expansion. This has many causes, but its net effect is a population that constantly augments through a sustained birth rate and a decrease in child deaths. About half of the population in this area is under 15 years of age. The United Nations has estimated the following figures for the years to come (cited in Anzola, 1985). Life expectancy at birth is anticipated to increase from 64.1 years in 1980-1985 in both Latin America and the Caribbean, to 71.8 in Latin America and 70.7 in the Caribbean in 2000-2025. In the same years the number of people (in thousands) is expected to enlarge from 363,704 to 865,198 in Latin America and from 30,648 to 61,887 in the Caribbean. The number of people above 60 years of age is predicted to gain from 23,328 to 93,317 in the whole Region. This is truly an "elderly boom," since the general population increase will be of 237% and that of the elderly 400%! This age group will become 10.8% of the population.

This situation has a series of consequences. The health of the elderly is worse than that of their younger cohorts since they tend to have more chronic and degenerative diseases as a result of their age. This creates demand for more medical services and for growing numbers of members of the health team, specialized in geriatrics. Some old people are bedridden and need hospital care. At the same time, the enlargement in the number of the elderly with the decrease of men and women who are economically active will be a burden to the social security systems of the Region, that will have proportionally less resources for a larger population. Money will also be increasingly spent in paying for pensions and disabilities.

Migration

Several countries of Latin America and the Caribbean suffer the "megalopolis syndrome." This means that they have few large cities and a host of scattered small towns, villages, and hamlets. One of these large cities is usually the capital, where one can find most of the administrative structure of the country, large industries, centers for higher education, medical care, and the best places for leisure, among many sources of income and public need or attraction. On the contrary, rural areas tend to have less public services, education, sources of income, social stimulation, and are poor and isolated. Better transportation has favored the possibility of migrating from rural areas to the larger cities.

The consequence of this situation is that urban areas grow larger, and the rural areas become depopulated. People go to the big cities thinking that they offer better opportunities. They settle in the marginal areas, creating the squatter settlements that are known in Latin America under names such as *barrios nuevos*, *asentamientos precarios*, *villas miseria*, *ciudades perdidas*, *favelas*, etc. This internal migration has complex results. There is a large pressure to create sources of income in the cities, rural food production diminishes, many people work in the area of services and not in the primary production of goods, the national budget becomes burdened by governmental investments in providing services to this increasing population, etc. But probably one of the most important results is that the population abandons its traditional culture, to adopt the urban pattern, which is usually a form of the so called Western cosmopolitan way of life. In many cases this gives rise to hybrid cultures in which tradition and modernity overlap, but there is a definite change in the values and in the lifestyle of people.

In some countries the situation is made more complex due to the possibility of migrating legally or illegally to a more affluent country. This is the case of the extensive exodus from Central America, Mexico, and the Caribbean to the United States, the migration of Central Americans to Mexico, of Bolivians to Peru, Colombians to Venezuela, and many others. The explosive political situation of several countries in the area has favored this international movement. Its effects are again very intricate, but among them, one can find: (a) the flow of foreign and usually harder currency to the family that has been left behind; (b) the breaking of family ties, due to the migration of young adults that leave behind their children and their elders; (c) the importation of different lifestyles and values, such as electronic and electric gadgetry, food, vehicles; (d) the desire to live as they do in other countries; and many others.

Social and Political Upheaval

This Region has been socially and politically unstable for a long time. Its revolutions and war take a toll on the whole population but mostly among the young. Sometimes the elderly are left without support, many women become widows or do not have the possibility of finding a stable companion. Social and political upheaval contributes to migration. This situation affects the whole social structure, increasing the numbers of the elderly, particularly of women.

CULTURE AND THE CARE OF THE ELDERLY

Despite the cultural complexity of Latin America and the Caribbean, it can be said that the traditional ways of life are being substituted by modernization and cosmopolitism. This has changed the attitudes towards the elderly and their care.

In general, traditional societies have reverence for old people. They are considered as ancestors, sources of wisdom, teachers, moral examples, the link of the living with the deceased, and in some cases they are attributed supernatural powers. For instance, the Nahuatl-speaking people that lived in Central Mexico before the arrival of the Europeans supposed that the *tonalli*, one of the three souls of man, became stronger as time passed and people acquired social positions and experience. They were also conscious that old people could have mental deterioration and become an *oppa piltontli*, or child for a second time (López Austin, 1980). In many societies there is a sense of responsibility for the care of the aged. Usually this is done within the family. Sometimes this is the natural result of life. Men, and particularly women who do not marry will tend to continue living with their parents. This is frequent when access to land for cultivation is gained by forming part of a household, and where housing is scarce. On the other hand, in societies where married couples leave their parent's home to establish their own, it is usual for the eldest daughter to invite one of their parents to live in her house, when the other partner dies. It is also true that grandchildren are "loaned" to the household of the elderly who are alone or handicapped. These situations are common in villages where families live together and where the living conditions are not too challenging. In stressful conditions it has been reported that the elderly who are not self sufficient die of neglect.

According to information that has come from research done in Latin America, it can be stated that the aged have a high status where society: (a) is socioeconomically homogeneous, (b) has sequential roles that entail progressively higher responsibility and authority (such as the *cargo* system of civil and religious authorities, not linked to the official government, found in the Region, (c) has a life-cycle sequence of roles characterized by continuity, (d) allows the elderly to control important family or community resources, (e) permits old people to engage in valued, useful, and important activities, and (f) where the extended family is a viable residential or economic unit (Finley, 1981 and Press et al., 1972).

The socioeconomic changes that go with urban lifestyles have modified the care of the elderly. Cities have among others the following characteristics that affect this situation: (a) higher population density, (b) costly living, (c) a more difficult access to food, (d) a rigid time schedule due to the type of employment found in them, (e) less physical security, (f) the need to use some kind of transportation, due to difficulties to move to and fro, (g) isolation due to the size of cities and the cost and problems associated with transportation, (h) crowding, and many others. The pressures of life in the cities cause nuclear families to become isolated and to give less and less support to the elderly. Young people are more likely to migrate into cities and leave their parents in the rural areas where they come from. Once in the cities young people try to find places to live by themselves and consider their parents and grandparents a burden. This has created the need of special institutions to keep old people. Some of them need hospitalization because of their senility, chronic diseases, or lack of capacity for self-maintenance. Unfortunately, in poor countries this is not always possible and old people suffer and are abandoned. This is particularly tragic in cases of persons who have no family. Of course this situation is not the same among all socioeconomic levels. The affluent have access to nursing homes and can pay servants or nurses to take care of their parents. Persons who are covered under the social security systems that exist in the Region receive social and economic benefits. Among them, is an economic pension, usually at or below the minimum wage, access to medical care, possibility of hospitalization in case of acute or chronic diseases, etc.

In Latin America and the Caribbean churches may play a very important role in the care of the elderly. These are places where they feel comfortable and find the social atmosphere that allows them to interact and provide activities that help people cope with the daily problems of life. For instance, many churches sponsor nursing homes or home visits for people who need them. The Catholic Church plays an important role in these matters through several of its orders of nuns and friars. What one does not frequently find in these countries are services such as the delivery of hot meals at home, or day care centers, but these are starting in some areas.

It is important to stress that Latin America and the Caribbean are very heterogeneous in the way that they treat the elderly. One can find groups with very simple technology and a social organization that some consider primitive, such as the Indian tribes of the Amazonian of Central American forests. In contrast, the Region also has some of the most populated and cosmopolitan cities such as Rio de Janeiro, Buenos Aires or Mexico City.

SOME DATA ABOUT FAMILY CARE
OF THE ELDERLY

The literature about family care of the elderly is scanty. Very few articles or books deal exclusively with this matter. Information can be found in texts dealing with other aspects related to this age group. In addition, research done in Latin America and the Caribbean is scattered in hard to find journals and books. In the following paragraphs appear some examples of the family care of the elderly, found in the literature.

Santo Tomás Mazaltepec is a *Zapotec* community in the valley of Oaxaca, Mexico. Its inhabitants speak their language in daily life and some use Spanish in transactions with people who do not speak Zapotec. It is a small and isolated village of about 1,245 persons. People are poor, they grow corn, and are subsistence farmers with no other important sources of income. Mazaltepec can be considered typical of the many Indian communities in Southern Mexico and Central America. In regard to the care of the elderly, one striking fact is that they are not isolated. They tend to live in three generation households; for instance, about half of the men and 90% of the women of 50 or more years of age have their grown children living with them. A very small minority of the elderly live alone. If they do not share their household with their children, they do it with their siblings, parents-in-law, or even with people who are hired to help them in their tasks as farmers. About half of the children from 13 through 17 years of age in the village live with their grandparents, although it would seem that they would be the least likely to do so. Some grandchildren either choose to or are sent to live with their grandparents to keep them company. The elderly are well informed of the gossip of their village; they are a very active part of their society. Death is seen as inevitable and it is customary for the whole family to be at the death-bed of the elderly. Nevertheless, the whole situation is changing with the contact of the Zapotecos with the values of urban life. For example, the knowledge of the elderly in the traditional ways has become less important; they do not know about the new technology or the "modern" ways of life, which are considered important by younger people. Even so, the elderly still have ways to keep their authority. Among them are their ownership of land and other possessions, which they can inherit or give away at their will. The expectations of younger people about this are controlled by the elderly in subtle ways, such as preferring those that have given them support in their old days, the ones who live with them, those who are more industrious and honest in their dealings, etc. Of course this form of social control works both ways. Sons and daughters who feel that their parents did not provide for them, will not feel responsible for the welfare of the elderly. This situation further being transformed now that the younger generations are finding other sources of income, as in the case of those who migrate to the cities (McAleavy Adams, 1972).

A similar situation is found in *Bojacá, Colombia*, a peasant village in the Andes. They are also poor subsistence farmers who are interested in reaching the level of the urban life of Bogotá, the capital. The elderly are much respected. They also tend to live in two generation houses and they also can have grandchildren on "loan" from their own sons or daughters. Old people are sought to help in specific tasks, such as cooking, going to the market, curing with medicinal plants, doing justice, counseling others about personal problems, religion, etc. But they are avoided when problems arise in the areas of economic activities that involve the exchange of cash or dealing with nonvillagers, the use of mechanical devices, formal education and school activities, village planning, romantic or sexual matters, etc. The advantage of being old in this town is that they know their place in society, and fulfill important roles and find positive reinforcement in their activities. As in the case of the Zapotec, this situation is changing (Kagan, 1980).

Costa Rica is one of the most developed countries in Latin America. It has shown considerable interest in the welfare of its aged population. Their life expectancy at birth is of 73 years. The situation of the elderly is similar to the one found in developed countries. Among 2,114 persons from 60 to 64 years of age, a third did not have a spouse; this figure increased to 62% among those over 75, and was higher among women. Out of 882 elderly that did not have a partner, 14.62% lived alone. The country has responded by creating several programs to improve the quality of life of the elderly. They have 32 institutions to house 1,944 old persons and 6 homes that offer aid to the disabled. The University of Costa Rica has created a program to allow the elderly to pursue studies (Brenes, 1987 and Trejos, 1985).

Uruguay also has an exceptional situation: it has a greater elder population than most countries in Latin America. Its life expectancy is high with a low birth rate. Young people tend to emigrate to other countries. The elderly are concentrated in urban centers. It has problems that are similar to those of developed countries: an increasing number of elder women who are left alone, a trend towards two generation households, loss of roles and few sources of income for the aged, etc. The government has tried to give social protection for this group, but their pensions are low and there are few facilities for their care (Alberieux, 1980). The social implications of this situation have been well explored (Ganón, 1970).

Seen as a whole, from the few data found in the literature, the situations in Latin America and the Caribbean seem to have a great deal of variability. It is important to state that health care delivery in the Region is provided basically by three types of institutions: governmental, private, and the social security systems. In regards to the care of the elderly, the three of them are well prepared to deal with acute illnesses, and the medical or surgical care of chronic problems. The government and social security systems provide pensions for those who have worked for a number of years or are disabled. But other types of care, such as nursing homes, day care centers, the provision of meals, etc. are left to the private sector and in most cases to the church. The majority of the community based services for the elderly consist of nursing homes, which range from the traditional poor ones, to the newer and modern, destined to the affluent sectors of society. There is also a growing number of clubs and organizations that gather the elderly together and in some countries sponsor specific organizations to handle their global problems (Tapia Videla, 1982). The situation has not improved as it would be desirable, due among other things to the political and economic instability of the Region.

PRELIMINARY RESULTS OF A SURVEY

Precise knowledge about the situation of the elderly is needed in order to develop a regional strategy for the care of their problems. As seen in the last section of this chapter, the information is meager and irregular. This is the reason why the Pan American Health Organization has started a survey on the needs of the elderly in selected Latin American and Caribbean countries. This survey is still in process and the data that will be presented here are to be considered preliminary and tentative, since they are based only on partial results. The importance of this survey is that it is being applied with the same content and methodology in different places of the Region, and will provide a first "snapshot" of the situation of people over 60 years of age.

Trinidad and Tobago (PAHO, 1987a)

Trinidad and Tobago is one of the Caribbean countries included in the study. A sample of 875 persons of both rural and urban areas was interviewed.

As in most of the world, women live longer than men and widows were frequent, but at age 80, the number of men and women who have lost their spouse is about the same. The majority of the elderly lived within two to three generation households, but 13.6% lived alone. Most of the men lived with their wife, and both sexes shared their home with the family of one of their children and their grandchildren. More men than women owned their house; it was more frequent for women to live in a house that was not their own. About a quarter of men under 70 and women over that age, felt that the facilities found in their houses were inadequate. Most houses (70%) had electricity, a shower, and a stove. Drinkable water, a refrigerator, an indoor toilet, television, and radio were less frequent in this order; telephones were scarce (20 to 30%). There were differences of about 10% in these items between men and women. Very few people reported not having either an indoor toilet or an outhouse (2.3%). The average number of people who lived with the elderly went from 2.4 to 3.9, with more persons living with those of more advanced ages.

Most of the men under 80 and women under 75 called themselves healthy. Those who had health problems agreed that they had difficulties to carry out needed or desired activities. From 40 to 45% of those above 80 reported visual problems as creating problems in their life; less than 20% had disabilities due to hearing problems, and 15 to 35% had difficulties chewing their food.

Almost all of the elderly interviewed could complete the basic personal self care activities, such as dressing and undressing, combing their hair, taking a bath, using a toilet, walking on a flat surface, and taking their own medicine. Most of those under 80 could carry out more complicated activities as cutting their toenails, doing housework, cooking meals, or climbing stairs. These activities could be done by few of those over 80. A good number of the elderly needed help to venture away from their home. Men came out as more dependent than women for the care of their illnesses. In the case of married couples, the wife usually took care of her husband, but not vice versa. Sons and daughters were the most frequent source of help.

The greatest problem that the elderly perceived was economical, followed by health. These surpassed the need for health and social services, housing, transportation, family, isolation, and social rejection. One quarter of those men over 70 and women under that age reported that their housing needs were not adequately satisfied.

This survey concludes stating that more elderly over 80 years of age can be defined as needy, both in their health, physical functioning, and financial situation. Eighty years of age seems to be the threshold of a decline in the satisfaction of the basic needs of those interviewed. Those living alone after this age are in a particularly difficult situation.

Costa Rica (PAHO, 1986)

As mentioned before, Costa Rica is one of the most socially developed countries in the Region. Its population has a high coverage by the social security system, its rate of literacy is high, and its political and economical situation has been quite stable.

A sample of 1,156 persons was obtained. Of these, 59.7% was in the urban areas and the remainder was in the rural part of the country. As expected, many more women (32.4%) than men (10.8%) were widowed. Women became widows at earlier ages than men. Very few were divorced (2.1%). The average household size was 4.6 people. There were more persons living with those above 80 years of age in the urban samples. Most of the houses were of two or three generations, but some reached four generations, since they included great-grandchildren. Only 7.5% lived alone, and 13.3% were couples living alone. Most of the elderly owned their house or lived in one belonging to their family. In the urban areas from 6% to 16% rented their dwellings. Less women than men owned their houses, due to being widows and having moved to live with their family. As age increases, this becomes more important for both sexes. Seventy to 80% of the houses had drinkable water, electricity, toilet, bath or shower, stove, and radio. Many of them also had television and refrigerator, but in the urban areas only half of the houses had a telephone. A little less than a fifth of the rural and a third of the urban men between 60 and 64 received a pension. This figure increased to between 50 and 60% at latter ages, but it was always less among rural men and women in both areas.

About 80% of the sample considered their health as adequate, but about half of them felt that their health impaired them to accomplish what they needed or wanted to do. One quarter of the sample felt that their vision created problems; the figure is less than 2% for hearing problems. Both vision and hearing were more frequently reported as a problem after age 80. Dental ailments caused difficulties in feeding for 18.3%. About 86% of the sample said that they had right to receive medical care in a public institution. Only 10% more claimed this in the urban areas contrasted to their rural counterparts.

Nine out of ten elderly could bathe, dress, groom, feed themselves, get in and out of bed, and remain continent without help. Twenty percent of those over 80 could take their medicines by themselves, 40% could not do their house work, and 33% needed help preparing their food. Women were more likely than men to be able to prepare their own food. The most difficult activities for these elderly were climbing stairs, cutting their toe-nails, taking a bus and leaving the house. As in the case of Trinidad and Tobago, those aged 80 and over were more dependent than the younger ones. Most of the help comes from family members and more frequently from spouses and daughters. Health and economy were cited as the main problems in this sample. Rural elderly over 75 and urban women over 80 can be considered needy, particularly in their health and economic needs.

Chile (PAHO, 1987)

Chile is a country that has a varied population, ranging from isolated Indian tribes to cosmopolitan cities. The sample for this survey was taken only from urban communities of more than 100,000 inhabitants, where 80.1% of the Chileans live. The survey was answered by 1,562 persons.

One interesting aspect of the Chilean study is that the communities could be classified as old, transitional, and young. Old communities were those where more than 10% of their people were aged 60 or more. The percentage for transitionals was from 6% to 9.9%, and 5.9% or less for the young communities. The sample was analyzed separately for each type of community, but the number in the young ones was too small to be considered separately.

As in Trinidad and Tobago and Costa Rica, women tended to lose their spouse before the men did, and eighty years of age also was the beginning of a period of greater vulnerability for both sexes. Women were widows in a proportion of three to one, in relation to widowers. Less than 10% of the sample were divorced. Most of the elderly lied in two to four generation households; the average home of the transitional communities was larger than the one of the old ones. It was more frequent than men lived with their wife, than for women to live with their husbands, because of the high rate of widows. This also accounts for the larger number of men (20 to 30%) who lived isolated with their couple, in contrast with the women who did so (less than 25%). More people lived alone in the old communities (10.9%) than in the transitional ones (5.4%). Nevertheless, 12% of those between 75 to 79 years of age lived alone.

About two thirds of the sample lived in their own house; the rest lived in one owned by their family, but an important number lived in a rented dwelling. Nine out of ten homes had drinkable water, electricity, toilet, kitchen, radio, and television. In the old communities, bathrooms or showers and telephones were more frequent than in the transitional ones; but telephones ranged from 30 to 70% depending on the community.

Most of the sample under age 80 could take care of themselves, but more needed help to leave their homes and to climb stairs. Self care needed more help after 80 years of age. Help was usually provided by another family member, being this was more frequent in the old communities. One important finding in Chile is that one tenth to one fifth of the elderly of the old communities stated that they did not have any potential help if they would become ill. Daughters were frequently cited as a source of help by both men and women who did not have a living partner.

Most of the sample was satisfied with their economic situation. Most of the men had pensions; women depended on more varied sources of income. As in the two other countries, the most frequently expressed concerns were related to economy and health. As in the two other countries, the most frequently expressed concerns were related to economy and health. As stated in the two other countries, visual, hearing, and dental problems became more serious after age 80.

CONCLUSIONS

The analysis of the data from the literature and the preliminary results of the survey lead to the following conclusions:

1. The family care of the elderly in Latin America is highly variable. It goes from the total involvement of society in the welfare of the elderly in gerontocratic Indian groups, to the nearly complete isolation of some old persons in the large cities.
2. The death pattern of the sexes causes that men tend to be cared for by their wives, but once women become widows, their family, and particularly their daughters become responsible for their welfare.
3. There is a difference in the quality of life after age eighty, when people become more dependent on the help of others, due to the deterioration of their vision, hearing, chewing, and capacity for self care.
4. The group with a higher risk are women over 80 years of age that live in urban communities.
5. The different social organization of the family found in the countries of the sample affects the care of the elderly.
6. The generalized notion that children are a good investment for old

age holds true, according to the results of the survey. Daughters in particular take a more active role in the care of their parents.

7. The way a person acts through his lifetime, especially in relation to accumulation of material wealth, friendship, and love, determines in good part his situation as an old person.

8. The smaller the community in which the elder lives, the greater his chances are of finding help.

9. The larger the family of the elderly, the greater the possibilities of having someone to live with them. This included the cases of grandchildren "on loan."

10. In general the elderly of Latin America and the Caribbean fare relatively well, probably because they are the survivors of cohorts with high mortality in childhood and adulthood.

11. Most of the elderly can take care of themselves at home; they need more help to climb stairs, leave their homes and prepare their meals. This has consequences for the design of housing for them and the type of help that has to be planned.

12. Latin America and the Caribbean are in the stage when concern for the elderly has arisen. According to some studies (Teski, 1982), concern not necessarily means action and excessive concern may take the place of action. Thus, now that we have some of the basic information, it is time to proceed to carry out concrete programs to help the elderly. The number of elderly in the Region is not as overwhelming as it is in Europe or the United States. Governments need not wait for their number to increase to take definite steps. The time to do it is now.

REFERENCES

Alberieux Murdoch, Americo S. Uruguay. In Erdman Palmore (editor): *International Handbook on Aging. Contemporary developments and research*. Westport, Connecticut, Greenwood Press, pp. 455-466, 1980.

Anzola Pérez, Elías. El envejecimiento en América Latina y el Caribe. In, Organización Panamericana de la Salud: *Hacia el bienestar de los ancianos*. Washington, D.C., Organización Panamericana de la Salud, Publicación Científica 492, p. 9-24, 1985.

Brenes Blanco, Adelina. *Old age and its effect on the isolation of the elderly*. San José, Costa Rica, typed manuscript, January, 1987.

Finley, Gordon E. Aging in Latin America. *Spanish Language Psychology* 1:223-248, 1981.

Ganón, Isaac. Problemas sociales del envejecimiento. *Revista Mexicana de Sociología*, XXXII (1): 169-191, 1970.

Kagan, Dianne. Activity and aging in a Colombian peasant village. In Christine

L. Fry (editor): *Aging in culture and society. Comparative viewpoints and strategies*. New York, Praeger, pp. 65-79, 1980.

Kerns, Virginia. Aging and mutual support among the Black Carib. In Christine L. Fry (editor): *Aging in culture and society. Comparative viewpoints and strategies*. New York, Praeger, pp. 112-125, 1980.

López Austin, Alfredo. *Cuerpo humano e ideología. Las concepciones de los antiguos nahuas*. México, Instituto de Investigaciones Antropológicas, Universidad Nacional Autónoma de México, Serie Antropológica 39, pp. 319-328, 1980.

McAleavey Adams, Frances. The role of old people in Santo Tomás Mazaltepec. In Donald O. Cowgill and Lowell D. Holmes: *Aging and modernization*. New York, Appleton-Century-Crofts, pp. 103-126, 1972.

Mesfin, Elizabeth, Dinesh P. Sinha, Peter J. Justum, William K. Simmons and Denise Eldemire. *Nutritional status, socio-economic environment and the lifestyle of the elderly in August Town, Kingston, Jamaica*. Kingston, Caribbean Food and Nutrition Institute publication J-51-84, 1984.

PAHO: Needs of the elderly survey. *A profile of the Costa Rican elderly*. Health of the Adult Program, Health of the Elderly Subprogram, Pan American Health Organization, typewritten preliminary report, October 1986.

PAHO: Needs of the elderly survey. *A profile of the elderly in Trinidad and Tobago*. Health of the Adult Program, Health of the Elderly Subprogram, Pan American Health Organization, typewritten preliminary report, October 1987a.

PAHO: Needs of the elderly survey. *Perfil del anciano en Chile*. Health of the Adult Program, Health of the Elderly Subprogram, Pan American Health Organization, typewritten preliminary report, June 1987b.

Press, Irwin and Mike McKool Jr. Social structure and status of the aged, towards some valid cross-cultural generalizations. *Aging and human development* 3(4): 297-306, 1972.

Tapia Videla, Jorge I. and Charles J. Parrish. *Planning for the health care of the elderly in Latin America and the Caribbean: Issues and problems*. Paper delivered at the American Public Health Association Annual Meeting, Montreal, Canada, November 1982.

Teski, Marea. What can the Industrial World teach the Third World about aging? In Jay Sokolovsky (editor): Aging and the aged in the Third World. *Studies in Third World Societies* 22:23-42, 1982.

Trejos, Alfonso. Implicaciones psicosociales del envejecimiento de la población costarricence. *Revista de Ciencias Sociales de la Universidad de Costa Rica*, número 29:9-16, marzo de 1985.

Werner, Dennis. Gerontocracy among the Mekranoti of Central Brazil. *Anthropological Quarterly* 54(1): 15-27, 1981.

Chapter Two

Life Satisfaction and Peace of Mind: A Comparative Analysis of Elderly Hispanic and Other Elderly Americans

Jane W. Andrews, MHS
Barbara Lyons, MHS
Diane Rowland, ScD

Editor's Introduction

Andrews, Lyons and Rowland provide a review of data gained from a 1988 telephone survey of over two thousand Hispanic elders. Their discussion of the strengths and limitations of this methodology are commendable. Although *Clinical Gerontologist* is primarily oriented to the needs of clinicians, some previous issues have carried articles and reviews concerning methodological issues in research:

Jane W. Andrews is Research Associate, Barbara Lyons is Research Associate, and Diane Rowland is Assistant Professor, Brookdale National Fellow, all at the Department of Health Policy and Management, The Johns Hopkins School of Hygiene and Public Health, 624 North Broadway, Hampton House Room 453, Baltimore, MD 21205.

The authors are grateful to The Commonwealth Fund for making the collection of these data possible, to Westat, Inc. and Louis Harris and Associates, Inc. who conducted the surveys, and to Judith Kasper, PhD for her help in both designing the survey and interpreting the results. The views expressed reflect those of the authors and not necessarily those of The Commonwealth Fund Commission on Elderly People Living Alone or The Johns Hopkins University.

1985 III (3) 85, 85-86
1985 IV (2) 61, 78-79, 80
1987 VI (3) 83-84
1988 VII (3/4) 93-94
1989 IX (1) 31-44, 77-78
1989 IX (2) 80-81

The conclusions are important for mental health practitioners as well as academicians:

1. Hispanic aged, in general, have lower life satisfaction, and are more likely to feel lonely.
2. Health care and financial difficulties are major stressors, and Hispanics are more vulnerable to these difficulties.

The authors consider social service and public policy implications, as well as those for mental health practitioners.

INTRODUCTION

Today, one million of the nearly 30 million elderly people living in the continental United States are Hispanic (U.S. Bureau of the Census, 1986). While the Hispanic population is currently small relative to the total elderly population, it is growing twice as fast. The number of Hispanic elderly is expected to quadruple by 2020 (U.S. Bureau of the Census, 1986). This expected increase has significant implications for social policy because elderly Hispanics are disproportionately poor and likely to have been disadvantaged educationally and in the workplace (Commonwealth Fund Commission, 1989b). This translates into less adequate retirement benefits and a greater likelihood of poor health or functional status compared with the general elderly population. Life satisfaction and peace of mind and happiness are linked to one's life history, but also to control over one's current situation. To the extent that elderly Hispanics are not afforded the same choices and opportunities for control over their lives as other elderly Americans because of economic and social barriers, they are likely to lag behind in overall well-being.

As a follow-up to a 1986 Louis Harris and Associates survey of the general elderly population, the Commonwealth Fund Commission on Elderly People Living Alone sponsored a national survey of elderly Hispanics in 1988 in order to obtain a profile of Hispanic elderly people and identify differences between the Hispanic and general elderly population. This survey was designed to provide new information on Hispanics with regard to their economic, health and social circumstances. The survey, conducted by Westat, Inc., showed that although some Hispanics have shared in the prosperity afforded many elderly people in this country, a great number face a daily struggle, living on limited incomes and coping with poor health (Commonwealth Fund Commission on Elderly People Living Alone, 1989b).

This paper extends that examination by considering differences in the well-being of the Hispanic elderly compared to the general elderly population. First, general characteristics of the Hispanic elderly population are contrasted to the total elderly population to help define socioeconomic differences. Next, measures of overall life satisfaction and peace of mind and happiness related to financial and social difficulties are contrasted between the Hispanic and total elderly population using responses to comparable questions asked in the 1986 Louis Harris survey of the general elderly population survey and the 1988 Hispanic study. Finally, the subjective well-being of Hispanic elders is explored in greater detail using questions posed on the Westat survey.

DATA BASE AND ANALYTIC METHODS

The primary data base for the Hispanic analysis is the 1988 survey of elderly Hispanics commissioned by The Commonwealth Fund Commission on Elderly People Living Alone and conducted by Westat, Inc. This telephone interview survey of 2,299 elderly Hispanics provides estimates of a nationally representative sample of Hispanics age 65 and over living within telephone exchanges with at least 30 percent concentrations of Hispanic residents in three subuniverses in the continental United States: New England and the Middle Atlantic states; Florida; and the balance of the United States. The sample selection and survey procedures have been described in detail elsewhere, but will be highlighted here (Westat, 1989).

The sample selection and telephone interviews were conducted from August through October 1988, following a pre-test in mid-July 1988. The 48,183 households screened for elderly Hispanics were selected by random digit dialing and resulted in completed interviews of 2,299 elderly Hispanics. The interviews were offered in both English and Spanish, with 87 percent of the sample choosing to be interviewed in Spanish (Westat, 1989). Telephoning was viewed as a reasonable means of obtaining a Hispanic sample because Census data indicate that about 92 percent of elderly Hispanics live in households with telephones.

In order to permit comparisons to be drawn between Hispanic and all elderly people, the Hispanic survey questionnaire included approximately two-thirds of questions from the Commission's 1986 national survey of elderly persons conducted by Louis Harris and Associates. In addition, the Hispanic survey was expanded to include some additional measures of well-being and family support.

The Louis Harris survey of the general elderly population was commissioned by the Commonwealth Fund Commission on Elderly People Living Alone in 1986 to provide insights into problems facing elderly Americans in general and those who live alone specifically. This survey was also conducted by telephone, using random digit dialing and has been described elsewhere (Louis Harris and Associates, 1987). In order to obtain a large enough sample and oversample of persons age 75 and over, 22,572 households were screened. The screening effort yielded 3,963 households and 1,535 for the oversample. A total of 2,506 interviews were completed for elderly people age 65 and over, including 48 Hispanics throughout the continental United States. The survey results were weighted by age, sex, race, education, region, and living arrangement using the U.S. Census Bureau estimates for the noninstitutionalized elderly population of the United States. All interviews were conducted in English. Concerns about underrepresentation of the Hispanic elderly population led to the follow-up Westat survey of Hispanic elderly.

Comparative analysis of Hispanics and all elderly is based on questions related to socioeconomic characteristics, health status, life satisfaction, and peace of mind and happiness common to both the Hispanic survey and the 1986 survey of all elderly. To assess peace of mind and happiness, elderly people were asked about serious problems in their lives including financial difficulties, such as not having enough money or having too many medical bills, and social difficulties, such as loneliness, having to depend too much on others, and caring for a sick spouse or relative. The Hispanic survey collected additional information about serious problems related to being anxious or having too many problems or conflicts within the family which is also presented.

The Hispanic survey also collected detailed information on morale and subjective well-being that was not in the Harris survey, but is presented here to provide a more detailed assessment of the Hispanic elderly on these dimensions. To measure overall subjective well-being and morale of elderly Hispanics, a variation on the Bradburn Affect Balance Scale (ABS) was used on the Westat survey (Bradburn, 1969). The scale was modified by substituting "I am going to read you a list of ways people sometimes feel. In the last few weeks have you felt . . ." for "looking at your present situation, have you ever felt . . ." This modification was designed to obtain information on the respondent's current state of mind.

The ABS is used to capture stresses and strains faced by "ordinary Americans in the pursuit of their life goals" and is considered a means of assessing morale and subjective well-being (Bradburn, 1969). The ABS is based on responses to 10 short yes-no questions that reflect positive or negative affects. The ABS is the sum of five positive items, or "Positive Affects" (e.g., happiness, pleased about accomplishment, excited or interested in something) minus the sum of negative items, or "Negative Affects" (e.g., upset, restless, depressed, bored), plus a constant of 5. The Affect Balance Scale scores range from a minimum of 0 to a maximum of 10 (Kane and Kane, 1981). In this analysis, scores are reported according to the percent scoring on the low end of the scale (a score of 0 through 5), the middle of the scale (scores of 6 or 7) and the high end of the scale (scores of 8 through 10). Thus, a high score indicates that a person is likely to have a more positive sense of well-being than a low score.

Before proceeding several caveats should be noted that are related to the survey design and methodology. Although overall response rates to both surveys were high—80 percent overall for the detailed Hispanic interviews, and 74 percent for the detailed interviews of all elderly—those with severe physical or cognitive impairments who are unable to respond to phone inquiries will be underrepresented in both surveys. In addition, telephone surveys also underestimate those of lower incomes who are less likely to have phone coverage. Both of these groups are likely to have lower levels of life satisfaction. Thus, their exclusion is likely to result in underestimates of physical difficulties and mental distress. Second, all information is self-reported; survey constraints did not permit independent verification of responses. In some cases, individuals did not respond to specific questions; the number of the sample respondents is noted on the specific tables.

RESULTS

The results of our analysis of the 1988 Hispanic elderly survey and the 1986 Louis Harris survey of all elderly people reveal startling information about elderly Hispanic Americans (Commonwealth Fund Commission, 1989b). The Hispanic elderly population experiences multiple economic, health, and social vulnerabilities. In many cases, these problems may reflect deficits accumulated throughout life, related to lack of education, linguistic problems, low-paying jobs, and poor health status. However, they also reflect an inability to respond to current situations because of economic and social barriers. Because elderly Hispanics are disproportionately disadvantaged, they are more likely to experience lower levels of life satisfaction, as well as peace of mind and happiness compared to all elderly people. Measures of well-being are closely tied to these socioeconomic factors and must be evaluated in conjunction with them.

Socioeconomic Characteristics

There are approximately one million Hispanic Americans age 65 and over, representing about 3 percent of the total elderly population living in the continental United States. The elderly Hispanic population tends to be slightly younger and slightly more likely to be male than the total elderly population. In addition, elderly Hispanics are far more likely to live with others and less likely to live alone than all elderly. Further, they have received less formal education and have lower incomes than the elderly population as a whole. Finally, the Hispanic elderly population is more likely to be in fair or poor health than all elderly.

Analysis reveals that compared to all elderly, the Hispanic elderly appear to experience multiple disadvantages related to education and economic resources, health and functional status, and the ability to live independently (Figure 1). Elderly Hispanics are twice as likely to have an eighth grade education or less compared to all elderly people (73 versus 35 percent). Lower education levels combined with difficulty in speaking English leads to a greater likelihood of holding low paying jobs with no pension or health insurance benefits throughout life.

As a result, despite having worked hard for most of their lives, many Hispanics find themselves in old age without the means to maintain their independence. Twenty-two percent of elderly Hispanics live below the federal poverty level compared with 12 percent of all elderly. Living on an income this low may lead to worry about difficulty in making ends meet on a daily basis and the ability to respond to needs should a household or health emergency arise.

For elderly Hispanics, a substantial portion of the population experience health and long-term care needs and may not have adequate resources to meet these needs. Over half of elderly Hispanics report fair or poor health, in contrast to about one-third of all elderly people. Forty percent have functional difficulties with basic self-care activities compared with 23 percent of all elderly people. These health and long-term care needs are likely to aggravate economic and social problems and threaten the ability of Hispanics to live independently. Hispanic elderly are more likely to live with children, siblings, other relatives, or unrelated people than other elderly people. Although this pattern of living arrangement may in part reflect cultural differences, it may also be closely tied to

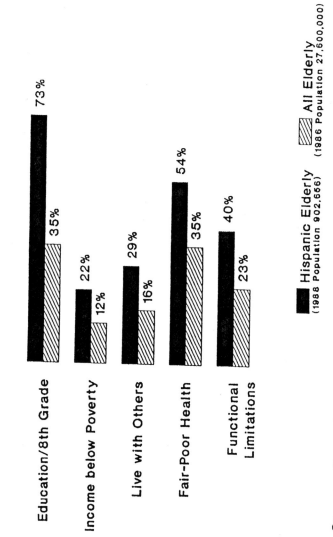

Figure 1: Hispanic Elderly Compared To All Elderly People for Selected Indicators

Education/8th Grade — 73% / 35%
Income below Poverty — 22% / 12%
Live with Others — 29% / 16%
Fair-Poor Health — 54% / 35%
Functional Limitations — 40% / 23%

Hispanic Elderly (1988 Population 902,656)

All Elderly (1986 Population 27,600,000)

Source: Commonwealth Fund Commission, 1989b.

an inability to cope without assistance related to low incomes and/or poor health and functional status.

The lower income and educational attainment levels of the Hispanic elderly population appear to result in greater levels of dependency and less ability for independent living and stable financial security. Worry about medical bills, delaying or foregoing medical care because of inability to pay, or having inadequate social support for oneself or other family members are all potential factors leading to lower levels of peace of mind and happiness among the Hispanic elderly. It is therefore likely that the Hispanic elderly population will experience less overall life satisfaction and more fears related to economic and social problems than other elderly people.

Life Satisfaction and Peace of Mind and Happiness

The relationship between socioeconomic factors and life satisfaction and peace of mind and happiness is striking for the Hispanic elderly population. Analysis of survey results shows that Hispanic elderly people enjoy less life satisfaction and are more likely to face serious problems, thus threatening the peace of mind and happiness they experience in their everyday lives.

General life satisfaction is lower among Hispanics than all elderly. Less than half of elderly Hispanics (48 percent) report that they are very satisfied compared with nearly two thirds of the general elderly population (62 percent) (Table 1). There is a dramatic relationship between health status and satisfaction with life, with poorer health status associated with more dissatisfaction. Among elderly Hispanics, only 22 percent of those in poor health report being very satisfied compared to 78 percent of those in excellent health.

Lower life satisfaction may also be related to having had lower educational attainment and lower paying jobs in the past, resulting in less adequate health and income benefits in retirement. Less than half of elderly Hispanics who had incomes in the past year of $15,000 or less reported that they were very satisfied, compared to 64 percent of those with higher incomes. These trends are similar to that for all elderly, although all elderly are slightly more likely to report being very satisfied with life.

The likelihood of facing serious problems in life that could undermine peace of mind and happiness is substantially greater for Hispanic elderly than all elderly (Figure 2). Elderly Hispanic Americans are far more likely to report serious problems related to financial and social difficulties than all elderly. For the types of problems examined, between 20 and 40 percent of the Hispanic elderly reported they experienced serious problems compared to seventeen percent or less for all elderly people.

Financial worries are a major source of concern for both Hispanic elderly and all elderly people, but the proportion of the population affected by this problem is much greater among Hispanics. Forty-one percent of elderly Hispanics report not having enough money to live on is a serious problem compared to 14 percent of all elderly. The likelihood of reporting lack of money as a serious problem is highest for those with low incomes, little education, and poor health status for both Hispanic and all elderly population groups, but the magnitude of the problem is much greater among the Hispanic population. Among those with incomes below about $5,500 per year, over half of Hispanic elderly report serious problems related to money compared to 29 percent of all elderly. Similar results are also found for those with little education — 45 percent of elderly Hispanics report too little money as a serious problem compared to 21 percent of all elderly. As mentioned earlier, lower wage jobs in their younger years have contributed to inadequate retirement benefits and a high level of poverty among elderly Hispanics in their later years. Not being able to make ends meet results in hard choices between paying the health care bills and buying food and other necessities and undoubtedly lowers peace of mind.

There is less difference between the population groups in poor health, 58 percent of Hispanics report money worries compared to 49 percent of all elderly. This finding highlights the financial difficulties that elderly people in poor health may experience as a result of gaps in Medicare's coverage, despite the fact that almost all elderly have Medicare (Commonwealth Fund Commission, 1987b). Elderly Hispanics are nearly twice as likely to report having too many medical bills as a serious problem as all elderly. About one-third of elderly Hispanics report the problem compared with 17 percent of the elderly population. This differential between Hispanic elderly and all elderly persists across all socioeconomic characteristics, but not by health status. As with financial concerns related to lack of money, for those in poor health, there is no difference between the Hispanic and general elderly population in the level of concern over medical bills, almost half of both groups experience serious problems.

Elderly Hispanics are also much more likely to experience serious problems related to social difficulties compared to all elderly (Table 2). The differential between elderly Hispanics and all elderly in the likelihood of experiencing these social problems is greater than for the financial difficulties mentioned above. Compared to all elderly, elderly Hispanics are

TABLE 1. Life Satisfaction Among Elderly Hispanics Compared with All Elderly by Selected Characteristics.

	Percent Who Say They Are Very Satisfied	
	Hispanic Elderly, 1988	All Elderly, 1986
Total	48%	62%
Age		
65-74	49	64 [a]
75+	48	64 [a]
Sex		
Male	50	63
Female	47	61
Living Arrangement		
Alone	51	59
With Spouse	49	65
With Others	46	55

Health Status		
Excellent	78	80
Good	60	67
Fair	37	48
Poor	22	35
Education		
8th Grade or Less	45	59
Some High School	50	58
H.S./G.E.D.	49	63
Any College	47	67
Income		
$5,500 or less	46	58[b]
$5,501 - 10,000	43	51[c]
$10,001 - 15,000	45	62
$15,001 - 25,000	63	67
$25,001 +	64	75

Source: Westat, 1989 and Louis Harris and Associates, 1987.

[a] Percents based on unweighted numbers.

[b] Income Level at $5,100 or less for all elderly.

[c] Income Level at $5,101-10,000 for all elderly.

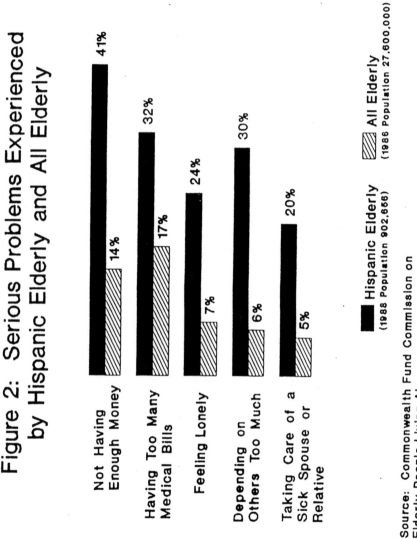

Figure 2: Serious Problems Experienced by Hispanic Elderly and All Elderly

Not Having Enough Money — 41% / 14%

Having Too Many Medical Bills — 32% / 17%

Feeling Lonely — 24% / 7%

Depending on Others Too Much — 30% / 6%

Taking Care of a Sick Spouse or Relative — 20% / 5%

■ Hispanic Elderly (1988 Population 902,666)

▨ All Elderly (1986 Population 27,600,000)

Source: Commonwealth Fund Commission on Elderly People Living Alone.

three times more likely to report loneliness or not having enough friends, five times more likely to report having to depend too much on others, and four times more likely to report having to take care of a sick spouse or relative as serious problems. Even when adjusting for socioeconomic characteristics, elderly Hispanics are much more likely to report these social problems than the general elderly population.

Overall, one quarter of elderly Hispanics report that loneliness or not having enough friends is a serious problem compared to seven percent of all elderly. The peace of mind and happiness of elderly Hispanics may be threatened since they not only have to cope with the attendant physical difficulties of poor health, but are also isolated from companionship outside the family. Living on limited incomes and being in poor health limits their ability to go out to meet people or participate in social activities. The inability to speak English may also contribute to isolation and loneliness. Interestingly, elderly Hispanics who are married or who live with others are about as likely to experience loneliness as elderly Hispanics who live alone.

Nearly one-third of Hispanic elderly report having to depend too much on other people as a serious problem. Elderly Hispanics are nearly twice as likely to live with others as all elderly (29 versus 16 percent) and often must live with others due to difficulties related to declining health and functional status or financial problems (Commonwealth Fund Commission, 1989b). Concern about having to depend on others too much within the Hispanic population may indicate that they may not be at ease with this living arrangement and feel that they are being burdensome to others. While some may assume that living with others has a protective effect on elderly Hispanics, it may in fact lower their peace of mind if the living arrangement is out of necessity and not out of choice.

One-fifth of elderly Hispanics report having to take care of a sick spouse or relative as a serious problem compared to five percent of all elderly. As expected, those who live with a spouse are more likely to experience this problem than other groups. It should be noted that as health status declines among the respondents, the percent reporting having problems related to taking care of a sick spouse or relative increases. This indicates that those who are having trouble providing care to the sick are themselves in poor health which may compromise their physical health and peace of mind.

For the most part, the likelihood of experiencing social problems appears to be more closely related to health status, education, and income than to age, sex or living arrangement. As health status declines, the per-

TABLE 2. Percent of Elderly Hispanics and All Elderly Reporting Types of Social Difficulties as a Serious Problem by Selected Characteristics.

Type of Social Difficulty Reported as a Serious Problem

	Percent Reporting Loneliness or Not Enough Friends		Percent Reporting Having to Depend too Much on Others		Percent Reporting Having to Care for a Sick Spouse or Relative	
	Hispanic Elderly 1988	All Elderly 1986	Hispanic Elderly 1988	All Elderly 1986	Hispanic Elderly 1988	All Elderly 1986
Total	24	7	30	6	20	5
Age						
65-74	23	6[a]	28	5[a]	21	5[a]
75+	25	8[a]	32	9[a]	19	5[a]
Sex						
Male	21	6	27	4	22	4
Female	26	8	32	7	19	6
Living Arrangement						

Alone	24	10	30	7	14	3
With Spouse	22	3	28	3	26	7
With Others	27	13	34	14	15	4
Health Status						
Excellent	13	3	19	1	12	2
Good	16	5	14	3	15	4
Fair	26	9	37	8	23	7
Poor	50	18	61	23	34	15
Education						
8th Grade or Less	25	9	32	9	21	6
Some High School	27	7	24	4	26	7
H.S./G.E.D.	17	6	22	5	17	4
Any College	14	4	18	3	14	3
Income						
$5,500 or less	30	9	38	13	24	6
$5,501 - 10,000	24	9	32	7	23	6
$10,001 - 15,000	22	7	26	5	19	6
$15,001 - 25,000	20	5	17	3	12	5
$25,001 +	13	3	15	2	10	2

Source: Westat, 1989 and Louis Harris and Associates, 1987.
[a] Percent based on unweighted data.

35

cent reporting serious problems related to loneliness, having to depend too much on others, and caring for a sick spouse or relative increases for both the Hispanic and general elderly population. Similar results are found with regard to lower education and income levels. The most vulnerable appear to be those in poor health for both Hispanic and all elderly people, however, elderly Hispanics are disproportionately affected. Among elderly Hispanics in poor health, 50 percent experience loneliness, 61 percent are too dependent on others and 34 percent report serious caregiving burdens.

Two additional measures of peace of mind are available from the Hispanic survey and include whether one experiences serious problems related to either being anxious or to having too many problems or conflicts in the family. Examination of these additional measures also shows that the Hispanic population appears to experience high levels of stress. Forty-one percent of elderly Hispanics reported being anxious or worried with concerns greatest among those who reported their health status as poor (Table 3). Poor health and functional status and low incomes among this vulnerable population are likely causes for anxiety or worry. Those with poor health status or who are economically or educationally disadvantaged are more likely to be anxious or worried.

Nearly a quarter of all elderly Hispanics reported having too many problems or conflicts in the family as a serious problem. Hispanic elderly in the younger age group, in poor health, experiencing functional limitations in activities of daily living, speaking Spanish only, and in the lower income groups were all more likely to say they had problems or conflicts in the family. Interestingly, those who live with others were the least likely to report this problem, perhaps indicating their dependence on family members.

Conflicts in the family appear to be more likely to arise if there are health and economic problems among elderly Hispanics. It is well known that illness in the family can cause stress and strain among family members. Thirty-five percent of those in poor health reported this problem compared with only 13 percent of those in excellent health. The proportion reporting this problem decreases as income increases. Only 11 percent of those in the highest income group reported family problems or conflicts as a serious problem compared with 27 percent of those in the lowest income group.

Subjective Well-Being of Elderly Hispanics

The survey of elderly Hispanics also provides insights into the subjective well-being and morale of this population, based on the Affect-Balance Scale (ABS). Living arrangement appears to have a protective affect on subjective well-being with high scores on the ABS indicating a more positive outlook on life. Elderly Hispanics who live with a spouse score higher on the ABS than those who live alone or who live with others (such as children or friends). Forty-four percent of those living with a spouse scored in the high group, compared with 34 percent of those living alone and 33 percent of those living with others (Table 4).

In addition, educational attainment and the ability to speak English as well as Spanish among elderly Hispanics has led to a more positive subjective well-being score. As might be expected, those in worse health and functional status were far more likely to score low on the ABS, indicating a more negative outlook on life. Finally, the differences in scores on the ABS according to income are striking. Seventy-nine percent of those with annual incomes above $25,000 scored high on the Affect-Balance scale, compared with about one-third (34 percent) of those below the poverty line. This finding is consistent with Bradburn's research showing those with higher incomes were more likely to have a more positive outlook (Bradburn, 1969).

DISCUSSION AND IMPLICATIONS

Elderly Hispanics face serious problems in their lives related to financial, health and social concerns. Compared to all elderly, elderly Hispanics are less likely to be very satisfied or achieve peace of mind or happiness. Elderly Hispanics are substantially more likely to report a number of serious financial problems, such as not having enough money or facing too many medical bills, and social problems, such as loneliness, being too dependent on others or having to care for a sick spouse. Those in poor health and those with low-incomes are particularly vulnerable. The higher the level of health status, income, facility with English, educational attainment, and functional status, the better the overall subjective well-being for elderly Hispanic people. Conversely, the lower the level of any of those variables, the lower the subjective well-being of elderly Hispanics.

These findings suggest several avenues for improving the overall well-being and peace of mind of elderly Hispanics. For health care practitioners serving the elderly Hispanic population, it is important to recognize that the well-being of elderly Hispanics is closely tied to underlying problems of poverty and poor health. In order to improve the peace of mind and subjective well-being of elderly Hispanics, it may be important to consider the social and economic problems facing elderly Hispanics. Practitioners need to examine the spectrum of needs of elderly Hispanics, whether it is improving financial protection or providing assistance with

TABLE 3. Percent of Elderly Hispanics Reporting Being Anxious or Having too Many Problems or Conflicts in the Family as Serious Problems by Selected Characteristics, 1988.

	Percent Reporting Being Anxious as Serious Problem	Percent Reporting too Many Problems or Conflicts in Family as Serious Problem
Total	41%	22%
Age		
65-74	44	24
75+	36	18
Sex		
Male	35	21
Female	45	24
Living Arrangement		
Alone	41	25
With Spouse	40	23
With Others	41	19

Health Status

Excellent	22	13
Good	28	18
Fair	49	25
Poor	70	35

Functional Limitations

Yes	56	28
No	31	19

Language

Spanish Only	46	28
English & Spanish[a]	37	19

Income

$5,500 or less	51	27
$5,501-10,000	38	22
$10,001-15,000	36	16
$15,001-25,000	29	18
$25,001 +	20	11

Source: Westat, 1989.

[a] includes those speaking English only.

TABLE 4. Subjective Well-Being of Elderly Hispanics Based on Affect-Balance Scale, 1988.

	Total	High (8-10)	Medium (6-7)	Low (0-5)
Population Estimate	722,575	281,804	267,352	173,413

		Percent Distributuion by Score [a]		
Total	100%	39	37	24
Age				
65-74	100%	40	37	23
75+	100%	36	38	26
Sex				
Male	100%	41	37	21
Female	100%	37	37	26
Living Arrangement				
Alone	100%	34	36	30
With Spouse	100%	44	35	21
With Others	100%	33	43	24
	100%			
Health Status				
Excellent	100%	59	33	9
Good	100%	45	42	14
Fair	100%	31	38	29
Poor	100%	19	25	55
Functional Limitations				
Yes	100%	26	35	39
No	100%	46	39	16
Education				
8th Grade or less	100%	36	39	26
Some High School	100%	38	34	28
H.S./G.E.D.	100%	48	36	16
Any College	100%	50	32	19
Language				
Spanish Only	100%	35	38	27
Spanish & English	100%	41	37	22

Income

- - - - - -

$5,500 or less	100%	34	36	30
$5,501-10,000	100%	37	41	22
$10,001-15,000	100%	43	36	21
$15,001-25,000	100%	55	24	21
$25,001 +	100%	79	16	6

Source: Westat, 1989.

[a] Percent Distribution Based on weighed estimates of sample responding to to scale questions.

health and functional difficulties. Clinicians can help to inform elderly people about the benefits of program enrollment and encourage people in need to apply to the program. In many states, enrollment in SSI automatically entitles one to Medicaid which could provide important assistance with the cost-sharing associated with Medicare, as well as other important health and long-term care benefits.

The Medicaid program can provide vital assistance with medical bills for low-income people. Medicare does not adequately cover medical expenses for elderly persons, but Medicaid provides assistance by filling in the gaps in Medicare and assisting with deductibles and cost-sharing for poor elderly people (Commonwealth Fund Commission, 1987b). As with the SSI program, many people who are potentially eligible for Medicaid are not aware of the benefits of participating in the program. The eligibility guidelines are complex and vary by state. Although nearly one-quarter of all elderly Hispanics live below the poverty line, only 44 percent of elderly Hispanics who are poor are enrolled in Medicaid (Commonwealth Fund Commission, 1989b). Clinicians should encourage elderly Hispanics to find out about and enroll in the Medicaid program. Expansion of Medicaid assistance to both the poor and near-poor elderly population would provide needed assistance and remove the fear of financial impoverishment from medical bills from the lives of many Hispanic elderly.

Better coverage of long term care services in the home for those with severe disability would serve the dual purpose of reducing the risk of impoverishment due to long term care expenses and promoting independent living in one's own home and reduction of the burden on caregivers (Commonwealth Fund Commission, 1989a). This would help to address the caregiving burdens and fear of dependence that trouble so many Hispanic elderly people.

It is also important to note that elderly Hispanics may not be "mainstreamed'' into society and some of the social status and subjective well-being indicators are in fact reflecting that lack of assimilation. Those who work with elderly Hispanics should consider cultural, educational, and linguistic barriers that may be present in the caregiving environment and try to facilitate care that is sensitive to cultural differences. Such efforts would help promote improved access to care and less anxiety related to medical care use. While this examination has provided some striking contrasts in life satisfaction and peace of mind between Hispanic elderly and the general elderly population, further research is warranted. Multivariate research analyses, including clinical studies, on the interaction of socioeconomic and health status variables on life satisfaction, peace of mind and subjective well-being are critical to designing practical interventions. Any combination of the efforts outlined above to improve public policy and greater research and clinical attention to the needs of the Hispanic elderly would go far in protecting the well-being of elderly Hispanics today and in the future.

REFERENCES

American Association of Retired Persons, Consumer Affairs. 1988. *Supplemental Security Income Demonstration Outreach Project: Final Report to the Commonwealth Fund Commission on Elderly People Living Alone.*

Bradburn, N.M. 1969. *The Structure of Psychological Well-Being.* Chicago: Aldine Publishing Company.

Commonwealth Fund Commission on Elderly People Living Alone. 1989a. *Help at Home: Long Term Care Assistance for Impaired Elderly People.*

The Commonwealth Fund Commission on Elderly People Living Alone. 1989b. *Poverty and Poor Health Among Elderly Hispanic Americans.*

The Commonwealth Fund Commission on Elderly People Living Alone. 1987b. *Medicare's Poor: Filling the Gaps in Medical Coverage for Low-Income Elderly Americans.*

Commonwealth Fund Commission on Elderly People Living Alone. 1987a. *Old, Alone and Poor: A Plan for Reducing Poverty among Elderly People Living Alone.*

Kane, R.A., R.L. Kane. 1981. *Assessing the Elderly: A Practical Guide to Measurement.* Lexington, Massachusetts: D.C. Heath and Company.

Louis Harris and Associates. 1987. *Problems Facing Elderly Americans Living Alone.* Report for The Commonwealth Fund Commission on Elderly People Living Alone.

U.S. Bureau of the Census. 1986. Current Population Reports, series P-25, no. 995. *Projections of the Hispanic Population: 1983-2080,* by G. Spencer.

Westat, Inc. 1989. *A Survey of Elderly Hispanics.* Report of the Commonwealth Fund Commission on Elderly People Living Alone.

SECTION TWO:
THE FAMILY CONNECTION

Chapter Three

The Family and Its Aged Members: The Cuban Experience

Gema G. Hernandez, DPA

Editor's Introduction

This section includes several chapters which focus on the role of family ties with Hispanic aging. From the role of conjoint couples counseling to intergenerational considerations of caregiving, family topics have been covered frequently by articles and clinical comments in *Clinical Gerontologist.*

1982 I (1) 69-86, 87-95
1982 I (2) 59-67
1983 I (3) 94-95
1983 I (4) 53-67, 75-76, 77-78
1983 II (1) 61-62
1984 II (3) 15-23
1984 III (2) 5-10, 11-17, 37-38
1985 III (3) 3-15
1985 III (4) 17-34
1985 IV (2) 19-30
1986 IV (4) 42-45, 47-50
1986 V 7, 24, 65, 97, 266, 268, 333-395, 417, 425, 429, 503

Gema G. Hernandez is Associate Professor, Nova University Institute for the Study of Aging, 13300 S.W. 108 Court, Miami, FL 33176.

I am indebted to my husband, Luis M. Hernandez, for his support and valuable assistance, and very appreciative to Miami Jewish Home and Hospital for the Aged, Channeling Project, specifically to Mary Guthrie, Sol Barquero, and Bill Collins.

1986 VI (2) 32, 56, 75-77, 85-97, 111, 113-119, 155, 158, 163,
    168-169, 173-175, 179
1987 VI (3) 67-70
1987 VI (4) 25-34
1988 VII (3/4) 109-125, 127-136, 63-166
1988 VIII (1) 71-73
1988 VIII (2) 43-62
1989 VIII (4) 51-53
1989 IX (1) 31-44, 45-52, 58-61, 64-67
1989 IX (2) 61-64
1990 IX (3,4) 1-18, 132, 147
1990 X (1) 3-15, 45-47, 48-51
1990 X (2) 17-34

Books on these topics have been frequently reviewed.

1982 I (2) 88
1983 I (3) 104-106
1983 I (4) 88-89
1983 II (2) 70-71
1984 II (4) 88-89
1984 III (1) 86-871985 IV (1) 73-75
1986 IV (4) 60-61, 65-66, 74-75
1987 VI (4) 85-86
1987 VII (1) 82-84
1990 X (2) 104-105
1991 X (3) 90-91

Hernandez considers one specific Hispanic group (Cubans residing in the U.S.) in order to identify its idiosyncrasies and the ties to historical-cultural experiences: African heritage, hierarchical structure of the family, guilt-induction, religion, overprotectiveness, and the socio-political background of the Castro Revolution. Specific suggestions are given to clinicians working with Cuban families with aged members.

In order to identify and deal effectively with mental distress among ethnic elderly, gerontologists and mental health specialists need to take into account the individual's cultural and linguistic context. Specific information about cultural values and beliefs of frail elderly Cubans and their elderly relatives, some of whom may or may not be their caregivers, are almost non-existent, even though the number of elderly Cubans is dramatically increasing. This chapter intends to fill a void, first by interpreting mental distress among ethnic elderly from their own cultural perspective, and secondly, by dealing with a target population which has not been the subject of much investigation: elderly Cubans and their caregivers.

CUBA: CULTURAL CHARACTERISTICS OF THE POPULATION

To understand Cubans, one needs to first understand the geographical location of the island and the dynamic fusion of the elements which created the present culture. Fusion from groups from the Iberian Peninsula (white population), and fusion of groups from Africa (black population) formed the basis of the Cuban culture which became the culture of integration, a *mestizo* par excellence (Saruski & Mosquera, 1979), an excellent example of syncretism (Sandoval, 1984), a culture that came to be known as the Afro-Cuban culture (Ortiz, 1942; Bustamante & Santa Cruz, 1975; Bernal, 1982). These influences, coupled with the unique relations between Cuba and the United States, explain the uniqueness of Cuban cultural traits and the Cubans' mode of adaptation (Sandoval, 1984).

It is this Afro-Cuban culture that teaches Cubans to respect their elders, follow their folk healing beliefs and *Santería* practices (Sandoval, 1984), use humor known as "choteo" as a defense function in the social reality of their culture (Manach, 1955), direct their activities to the "present" (Szapocznik, Scoppetta, Arnalde, and Kurtines, 1978), and orient themselves mainly to people or persons rather than objects or ideas (Szapocznik, Scoppetta, Arnalde, & Kurtines, 1978).

An important characteristic of the Cubans is their "familism" (Szapocznik, Scoppetta, Arnalde, Kurtines, 1978). The bond and loyalty Cubans have to the nuclear family, to the extended family, and the networks of friends and neighbors (Bernal, 1982) represents an important support and mediator when dealing with mental health issues as well as caregiver responsibility (Vitaliano, Maluro, Ochs & Russo, 1989). On the other hand, this represents a tremendous source of emotional burden mainly verbalized in the form of guilt feelings if an individual is not able or willing to fulfill his/her culturally prescribed caregiver role within a family unit. Familism began to disintegrate as a result of political ideology or family geographical separation. This is an important issue to identify early in treatment. If the family has been divided for political reasons or as the result of the migratory waves, mental distress could be the result, due to unresolved conflict occurring at the time of separation. Chances are a connection exists between the time migration to the United States occurred, or the reason for migration, and mental distress (Gonzalez-Reigosa, 1976; Bernal, 1982). Identifying and dealing with this unresolved conflict is the key to effective treatment.

Another factor to be considered is the hierarchical structure that exists within the Cuban family (Szapocznik, Scoppetta, Arnalde & Kurtines, 1978), determining which member of the family should be the caregiver for a frail relative. Traditionally, the role of caregiver is given to females; and within the female family members, it is given to the one with the lowest status. The family lineality starts, or is always headed, by the oldest married male and ends with the youngest unmarried female (Szapocznik, Scoppetta, Arnalde & Kurtines, 1978). When the hierarchy is not followed, family tensions emerge, creating psychological distress experienced by the person who is not fulfilling his/her prescribed family role. It is also felt by the person who is being forced to fill the vacant caregivers' role, and the frail elderly in need of care who feels rejected by the family, even though someone else is caring for him/her.

As a group, Cubans value verbal expression (Bernal, 1982). It is highly recommended that the therapist or gerontologist be able to communicate in Spanish, otherwise, the practitioner will miss the emotional content of the conversation and subtle comments which will show the "real" meaning of what is being communicated. These subtle comments can be linguistically translated but cannot be culturally translated. In addition, the practitioner will not be able to understand paraverbal channels of communication in the form of pitch, tempo, and intensity of the verbal exchange (Schnapper, 1981).

The Spanish language is probably one of the most important aspects of Cuban family life (Bernal, 1982). The family's degree of bilingualism will, in itself, tell the mental health specialist a great deal about potential family conflicts that could exist between the children, parents and grandparents. Pressure to succeed economically has pushed the younger generation of Cuban-Americans to "Decubanize" (Gonzalez-Reigosa, 1976; Bernal, 1982). Because of what the Cubans have accomplished in just 31 years, Perez (1976) Gonzalez-Reigosa (1976), Bernal (1982), and Pedraza (1990), and others, have concluded that as a group, Cubans have experienced overassimilation to the host culture. This overassimilation is creating a high degree of intergenerational conflict (Szapocznik & Herrera, 1978). The elderly Cubans are no longer able to communicate, understand or participate in their grandchildren's life. They are, therefore, isolated within their existing family units and find comfort only in their cohorts.

Cuban culture, just like the Jewish culture, introduces guilt early in life (Herz, 1982). It is a way of reminding daughters, and sometimes sons, that they are responsible for their parents and that these obligations should never be forgotten. With the "Decubanization" process that has taken place (Gonzalez-Reigosa, 1976), this mechanism is no longer working, and is further contributing to the mental distress experienced by the elderly population because they are no longer able to "control" through guilt the behavior of the younger generation.

Another important component that plays a role in creating or diminishing mental distress among elderly Cubans, is based on the values and beliefs they have learned from their Catholic upbringing which emphasizes the idea that we come to this life to suffer and to pay for our sins so we can go to heaven. Some caregivers that were part of the research project the author conducted from 1989 to 1990, saw a tremendous importance in their role as caregivers because the burden they were experiencing now was allowing them the opportunity to "pay for their sins" in this life. Other elderly relatives who decided not to take the caregiver role experience guilt and anguish over their decision.

It is crucial for the practitioner to understand the role of women within the Cuban culture in order to fully appreciate the changes they have gone through, as well as understand the importance of the role of caregiver within that cultural context.

The traditional role of a Cuban female was to keep the family together and to emulate as much as possible the Virgin Mary (Szapocznik, Scoppetta & Tillman, 1978). A Cuban woman was fearful to God, devoted to her children, faithful to her husband, and obedient to her parents (Szapocznik, Scoppetta, Arnalde & Kurtines, 1978; Bernal, 1982). The woman's own wellbeing was unimportant. Instead, what was important, was the wellbeing of others: her parents, her husband, her children, and her grandchildren.

One of the major sources of psychological stress comes from situations whereby the care recipient, usually an elderly grandparent, competes with the caregivers' children, his/her own grandchildren, for the attention of the caregiver, daughter/mother. Cuban women caught in situations like that, experience extreme guilt because they cannot perform simultaneously more than one of three culturally prescribed roles: mother/daughter/spouse. In all three roles, providing care to another person is one of the components.

Among old Cubans, women's roles outside their home is insignificant.

However, within the Cuban family, women have a central and controlling factor (Pedraza, 1990). They are responsible for the day-to-day operations of the home and make basic decisions about the destiny of the family. Marriage, home and family are their ultimate achievement (Szapocznik, Scoppetta, Arnalde & Kurtines, 1978).

Cuban women enter into marriage, generally speaking, in their late teens or early twenties with the expectation that their spouses will take care of them financially. There has been a noticeable tendency among Cuban women to marry much older men who can support them financially and can "mold" her to his likes and dislikes (Pedraza, 1990).

Paradoxically, Cuban men enter marriage with expectations that their spouse will take care of them, emotionally and physically, for the rest of their lives especially during their old age (Pedraza, 1990).

Cuban women are expected to educate the children and place their children's wishes and desires ahead of their own. It has been found that one of the primary jobs of the Cuban women is to encourage whatever talent the children have; therefore, she finds herself deeply invested in the accomplishments of her children. Cuban women are beginning to experience conflicting demands; people are now living longer and with extended longevity, her duty as a daughter conflicts with her primary job as a mother, educating and taking care of her children. In some cases, the above conflict increases due to the lack of connection with their natural supports in Cuba. Taking care of her elderly parents is posing tremendous physical, emotional and financial burden on her. How she is dealing with this burden was the main purpose of our research.

Within the Cuban culture, women express love in an indirect fashion. Love is demonstrated by the constant feeding of children, cleaning of the house, clothing of the children or loved one and general overprotective behavior toward the children of both sexes. This expression of love has continued among the elderly Cubans and is also being observed in the way a woman behaves as caregiver for her elderly spouse or elderly parents. The elderly Cuban female is proud that her loved one does not have any decubitus ulcers and is clean and well fed. Their overprotectiveness of the people they care for places an additional "welcome" burden in a woman's life. This additional burden is in itself rewarding because it increases her status within her family and in the Cuban community at large.

Finally, women within the elderly Cuban community are also viewed as more "emotional" than men (Szapocznik, Scoppetta, Arnalde & Kurtines, 1978). If they express emotions in public, like crying, nervousness, "ataques," those emotions are acceptable. The cultural acceptance of their emotionalism allows them a mechanism to express some of the stress they are experiencing because of their frailty, or as a result of their care-givers' role. In addition, because this emotionalism is culturally expected, it may not indicate "true" emotional burden, but fulfillment of social expectations.

CUBA: SOCIOPOLITICAL BACKGROUND

Since 1959, nearly one million Cubans, equal to ten percent of the island's population, have migrated to the United States, and the number keeps increasing (Strategic Research Foundation, 1988). The Cuban migration possesses unique characteristics that set them apart from other Hispanic or Latino groups (Bernal, 1982); these characteristics have contributed to their relative financial and professional success. Cuban-Americans are the most affluent and best educated of the Hispanics (Naisbitt, 1990). They own an estimated 15,000 businesses, from 500 grocery stores to two dozen banks (Sewell, 1990). The influence of Cuban-Americans continues to grow among the 100 most influential Hispanic businesses in this country. Politically, there is one Cuban in the U.S. Congress, three in the Florida Senate, and eight in the Florida House of Representatives. In the metropolitan Dade County area alone, there are six Cuban mayors and several commissioners (De Varona, 1990). There are several Cuban movie stars, one Cuban has received a Pulitzer Prize, one Cuban is the Chief Economist for the United States Department of Commerce; one Cuban is the superintendent of one of the four largest school systems in this country, and another Cuban is the vice president and chief executive officer of the largest community college system in the United States. All the above gains have been achieved in only 31 years.

One question to ask is how much this success has affected the values, beliefs and language skills of the Cubans. The answer depends upon the age of the cohort in question and how old the cohort was at the time of migration to this country. For the purpose of our research, what the author considers to be the first Cuban cohort, those individuals who came to this country in their late forties or older and are now in their mid-sixties or older, have not experienced the degree of acculturation or even assimilation that has been experienced by the second cohort and all subsequent cohorts. Elderly Cubans have not lost the majority of the values and beliefs they had at the time they came to this country. The contrast between this lack of acculturation among elderly Cubans, the acculturation of their children, and the overacculturation of their grandchildren seems to foster mental distress among elderly Cubans.

The 1959 Revolution created an unparalleled migration to the United

States, with unique consequences. Large numbers of Cubans began leaving the island in 1959, and the inflow continues. It is important to recognize that not all the Cubans that came to the United States came for the same reasons, nor do they represent a monolithic group. Four distinct migratory waves have been identified (Amaro & Portes, 1972; Perez-Stable, 1981; Pedraza, 1990), each with its distinct characteristics and mode of adaptation. For the mental health practitioner, recognizing the differences is very important if an effective intervention and treatment is to follow.

The first wave of Cubans began in 1959, shortly after the Cuban Revolution took over the country. Some researchers feel this first wave ended in 1961, while others believe it lasted until 1965 (Bernal, 1982). The author considers the first Cuban wave to last from 1959 up to 1961; and the second — after the Bay of Pigs invasion, April 17, 1961 — from 1961 to 1965. The first group came on a voluntary basis to this country, but never intended to remain here (Amaro & Portes, 1972). This is very important in understanding Cubans' mode of adaptation and their present psychological needs. This first wave of Cuban immigrants left their country for political reasons on a voluntary basis, with the belief they would return within a year's time to their homeland, just like previous migrations had done (Pedraza, 1990). After the failure of the Bay of Pigs invasion, it became clear to the Cuban community that there was no way back to the island (Bernal, 1982). Their stay in the United States became an involuntary stay even though their migration was on a voluntary basis (Amaro & Portes, 1982). Portes identified this group as the "real refugees" (Bernal, 1982). This cohort has never accepted their new status as an ethnic minority group. The second wave of Cubans and all subsequent arrivals came here with the full understanding of the permanence of that migration. Subsequent migrations also reveal differences in the reasons given by Cuban immigrants for leaving the island.

The third wave began in 1965, and ended in 1973 (Bernal, 1982). During this time, the United States created the Freedom Flights in an effort to reunite the Cuban family; specifically, the parents of the unaccompanied children. The Family Reunification Program brought a large percentage of middle class, skilled laborers and still mostly women and white Cubans to this country (Bernal, 1982). This family reunification program reunited the family physically, but not psychologically. One of the main reasons adult children place their parents in nursing homes, a behavior unaccepted in the Cuban culture, appears to be connected to the way the family left the island: who was left behind, who came, why they came, who brought them to this country, and who was responsible for supporting them throughout the first years in the United States. The placement of a family member in a nursing home is interpreted in the elderly Cuban community as punishment for past behavior rather than as something needed because of special circumstances.

The fourth wave began in 1980, and has not ended, even though the numbers have drastically diminished. What precipitated this wave was the 1980 incident at the Peruvian Embassy in Havana, which led to the arrival of 125,000 Cubans to the United States (Unzueta, 1981; Bernal, 1982). This fourth wave was totally different from the previous ones (Unzueta, 1981). This group exhibited more difficulties in adapting to the American culture. It is anticipated that their acculturation process will follow a different path than that of previous migrations. An important feature is the fact that the so-called Marielitos, Cubans coming from the Port of Mariel in 1980 (Unzueta, 1981), were not welcomed with open arms by the Cuban population residing in the United States (Bernal, 1982). With a great percentage of the Marielito population familism was no longer part of their value system.

CLINICAL CONSIDERATIONS

The gerontologist or mental health specialist should explore the family migratory history, the degree of bilingualism among family members, the geographical location of the extended family, the existence of a caregiver, and the relationship of that caregiver to the care recipient. Special attention should be given to the degree of acculturation present as it relates to the prescribed role women have within the Cuban culture.

While the therapists conduct the preliminary assessment, they need to remember that Cubans are very private people (Bernal, 1982), and this needs to be taken into consideration when assessing the family dynamics. As a family, they will present an outwardly "together" image in front of the therapist. They will project the problem to the outside environment rather than accepting responsibility for the situation. The family is OK, and every individual member is OK, will be verbalized by everyone involved while at the same time they may cry and complain about the lack of attention they are getting from their adult children. A contradictory situation that could only be interpreted if we understand that they will never directly verbalize criticism of their loved one to a stranger.

The present Cuban family does not display a group approach to resolving family problems. The elderly cohort may experience an interdependence relation with the next cohort, their adult children, but the third generation, their grandchildren, are not actively involved in the care of their grandparents. This finding is different from what Ramon Valle has found among the Mexican-Americans living in California (Henderson, 1990). Valle observed that in a Mexican-American Alzheimer's support group, multiple generations participated in group activities, including young children. This indicates that the entire family, as a group, from the smallest child to the oldest, was part of the group approach tackling the problem the elderly relative faced. Our findings are similar to what Henderson has found among Hispanic caregivers for Alzheimer's patients in Tampa, Florida (Henderson, 1990); even though our population and Valle's population have lived in this country 31 to 41 years. The Cubans responded similarly to Henderson's population, a population that has been in this country much longer. This further supports the overassimilation theory previously discussed.

Family disagreements over political issues are still an important source of mental distress among elderly Cubans (Bernal, 1982). Some of them lack connections with their natural supports in Cuba. Others have not forgotten how the brother or the father stopped participating in family affairs because of differences in political affiliation. A third group feels abandoned by their relatives who migrated early, leaving them behind. All of the preceding factors play a role in the present family dynamics and need to be explored when dealing with identifying the family's developmental process.

In a clinical setting, elderly Cubans will tell therapists how they have learned to accept their "burden," either because they see this as their "fate," or they believe that, as sinners, they deserve to feel guilty, depressed, or anxious. Another explanation could be that one of the *Santería* gods is mad at them or not pleased with what they have done. Many of the elderly consider that to attempt to alleviate their condition is to defy the will of God, either their Catholic God or their *Santería* God. The fact that the culture has prepared Cubans for a high tolerance for suffering explains why the suicide rate among elderly Cubans is fairly small (Pedraza, 1990). It also explains the martyrdom attitude observed in some of the elderly Cubans. Removing this burden as the therapeutic goal is something they may not be willing to consider. One cannot infer that a person is experiencing psychological distress as a result of the responsibility of taking care of a frail elderly family member (Vitaliano, Maluro, Ochs & Russo, 1889). On the contrary, what our preliminary research indicates is that this could be the only positive experience that the caretaker is having and can constitute a tremendous source of pride and status. For elderly

Cuban females, feeling in control of her family's destiny is important. As a caregiver, this may be the only opportunity she has of being in total control of her destiny and her spouse's destiny.

Clinicians need to be aware that a Cuban female may consider herself a failure if she cannot keep her house clean. A referral to a home health agency can work miracles even though they may not culturally understand the role of the nurse's aid. It is important for the therapist to explain the nurse's aid's role. From the author's personal observation, it has been noted that frail elderly Cubans will go to the trouble of cleaning the house before their nurse's aid arrives even though the nurse's aid is supposed to take care of their personal care and homemaking needs. This behavior has also been observed as reported by Henderson with his Tampa Hispanic Caregiver's Group (Henderson, 1990). As previously stated, cleanliness is a very important cultural trait which is considered a way of showing love for the family. Referring frail elderly Cubans to a community in-home services program, while explaining to the individual that it is culturally acceptable for her/him to receive assistance in performing those duties, can help release the mental distress produced by not having a clean house or by accepting help in cleaning one's house.

Helping elderly Cubans develop or enhance their social support system is one of the most important intervention strategies the therapist can use (Henderson, 1990). Social systems act as modifiers, and will buffer the effects of psychological distress experienced as a result of family, physical or financial problems (Vitaliano, Maluro, Ochs & Russo, 1989; Henderson, 1990). In building this social support, it is important to consider individuals who share the same migratory experience. Chances are, mutual acquaintances will be found, and for Cubans, it is important to have the same circle of friends and acquaintances. This has the immediate effect of establishing trust and camaraderie.

As stated above, Cubans are very private people (Bernal, 1982). They will put up a front to keep family problems in the closet. They will give the therapist excuses as to why the children are not taking care of them, or why they do not live with their adult children. In some cases, illnesses, like Alzheimer's, can bring public humiliation to the family (Henderson, 1990). If this becomes common knowledge, others may assume the family has "tara" or bad blood because of the Alzheimer's (Henderson, 1990). In the case of illnesses like dementia, senility, mental disorders (Henderson, 1990), mental retardation, and sexually transmitted diseases like AIDS, total secrecy is maintained. These illnesses and the effect they have on the individual and the family are not discussed with strangers.

Finally, it is very important to understand the issues of dependence versus independence within the Cuban cultural context (Bernal, 1982), before the therapist can help clients establish certain treatment goals. Cubans believe that establishing an interdependent status is completely acceptable. Total independence is not approved of, nor is it taught by the culture. Complete dependence on family members, such as adult children or spouses, is welcomed and is not interpreted as pathology (Bernal & Flores-Ortis, 1982). Trying to change that interdependence or co-dependence could be fought by the patient and the family, resulting in withdrawal from treatment.

Group therapy and/or participation in support groups as a vehicle for dealing with mental distress is extremely helpful (Vitaliano, Maluro, Ochs & Russo, 1989), especially if members of the group belong to the same cohort (migrated approximately during the same migratory wave); this has been collaborated by other researchers like Bernal (1982) and Henderson (1990). When putting together support groups, it is important not to mix older females with older Cuban males. If Cuban males are members of the group, the group will become a social group and will fail to produce therapeutic results. Elderly Cuban women will assume passive roles, allowing the males to control the group activities. It is preferable that older Cuban females should be in all-female groups with people from their own cohorts.

Treating Cubans as one would treat other Hispanic groups or even other minority groups is not going to work because Cubans do not consider themselves as "Victims of Society," nor do elderly Cubans consider themselves a minority group. They have not lost their sense of peoplehood, even though it is acknowledged that the next cohort of Cuban-Americans have lost a great deal of their language skills, are reconsidering the importance of the extended family versus the nuclear family, and are losing their predominant Catholic beliefs and values.

BIBLIOGRAPHY

Amaro, N. & A. Portes, (1972). Situacion de los grupos Cubans en Estados Unidos. *Aportes*, *23*, 6-24.

Bernal, G. & Y. Flores-Ortiz (1982). Latino families in therapy: Engagement and evaluation. *Journal of Marital and Family Therapy*, *8*, 357-365.

Bernal, G. (1982). Cuban Families. In McGoldrick, M., K.J. Pearce & J. Giordano (Eds.). *Ethnicity and Family Therapy*, 187-205.

Bustamante, J.A. & A. Santa Cruz (1975). *Psiquiatria Transculhual*. Havana. Editorial Cientifico-tecnica.

DeVarona, Tony (1990). Cubans in Miami. *El Nuero Herald*, November 9, 1990.

Gonzalez, Reigosa, F. (1976). *Las Culturas del Exilio Reunion: Boletin del Institito de Estudios Cubanos*, 89-90, September 1976.

Grau, Ramon (1987). Operation Peter Pan: What we did to save Cuban children. *Miami Herald*, August 1987.

Henderson, J.N. (1990). Alzheimer's disease in cultural context. In Sokolovky, J. (Ed.). *The Cultural Context of Aging*. Borgin & Garvey Publishers, 315-330.

Herz, M.F. & J.E. Roson (1982). Jewish families. In McGoldrick, M.; K. Pearce & J. Giordano (Eds.). *Ethnicity and Family Therapy*. The Guilford Press, 365-392.

Hispanic Business Magazine (1989) (editorial). The five hundred most influential Hispanic businesses in the United States.

Manach, J. (1955). *Indagacion del Choteo*. Havana. Editorial Libro Cubano.

Naisbitt, John. Surging U.S. Hispanic population reshapes nation's complexion. *Trend Letter*, 9 14, July 5, 1990.

Ortiz, F. (1974). *Los Negros Brujos*, Havana, Coleccion Ebano y Canela.

Pedraza, T (1990). Cuban Culture—A presentation to the Miami Mental Health Association, Police Training Program, August 1990.

Perez-Stable, E.J. (1981). Cuban Immigration: A Socio Historical Analysis. Presentation, Miami, 1984.

Sandoval, M. (1984). Cuban Health and Mental Health Practices. Presentation to community nurses, South Miami Hospital, April 1984.

Saruski, J. & G. Mosquera (1979). *The Cultural Policy of Cuba*. United Nations Educational, Scientific and Cultural Publications.

Schnapper, M. Nonverbal communication and the intercultural encounter. In Wong, Z.H. Multicultural Training Institute Seminars. Training programs for effective practices with multicultural population. Cleveland, Ohio, September 1987.

Sewell, John (1990). Cubans in Miami. *The Gainesville Sun*, November 8, 1990.

Strategic Research Corporation (1988). Status of the Cuban Community Report, presented to Nova University, December, 1988.

Szapocznik, J.; M.A. Scopetta; M. Arnalde & W. Kurtines (1970). Cuban Value-Structure: Treatment Implications. *Journal of Consulting and Clinical Psychology*, 46, 961-970.

Szapocznik, J. & M.C. Herrera (Eds.) (1978). *Cuban Americans: Acculturation, Adjustment and the Family*. Washington, DC: Westview, 1980.

Unzueta, S. (1981). *The Mariel Exodus: A Year in Retrospect*. Metro Dade County, Office of County Manager, Miami.

Vitaliano, P.P.; Maluro, R.D.; Ochs, H. & J. Russo (1989). A model of burden in caregivers of DAT patients. In E. Light & B. Lebowitz (Eds.), *Alzheimer's Disease Treatment and Family Stress: Future Directions for Research*, 267-291. Washington, DC: Government Printing Office.

Chapter Four

Ethnocultural Themes in Caregiving to Alzheimer's Disease Patients in Hispanic Families

J. Neil Henderson, PhD
Marcela Gutierrez-Mayka, MA

Editor's Introduction

Henderson and Gutierrez-Mayka expand on the family caregiving theme introduced by Hernandez in the last chapter. These authors identify major ethno-cultural themes in Hispanic health belief systems (e.g., stigma of mental illness), and follow up with a quantitative survey, and illustrative cases. The conclusion is that caregiving is tied in with cultural definitions of sex roles: caregiving duties of a frail elder fall first on a daughter, then on a daughter-in-law. Younger cohorts are modifying these ethno-cultural themes.

INTRODUCTION

The demands of providing home care to dementia patients sufficiently tax the coping resources of many caregivers so that mental health intervention is a necessity (Zarit and Zarit, 1982; Morycz, 1985; Oliver and

---

J. Neil Henderson is Assistant Professor in Psychiatry, Principal Investigator of the project yielding this paper, and Ethnic Minority Specialist at the National Resource Center on Alzheimer's Disease at the University of South Florida's Suncoast Gerontology Center. Marcela Gutierrez-Mayka is a doctoral candidate in applied medical anthropology, Assistant in Research for this project and Ethnic Minority Specialist at the above named Center.

This project was sponsored by the Administration on Aging, the State of Florida, Department of Health and Rehabilitative Services; Aging and Adult Services; and the University of South Florida, Suncoast Gerontology Center.

Bock, 1985; Lichtenberg and Barth, 1989). Many caregivers are older adults whose need for effective delivery of mental health services has been specified for some time (Busse and Pfeiffer, 1977; Zarit, 1980; Silverman, 1987). Also, general mental health intervention with ethnic populations has received special attention regarding the clinical relevance of cultural sensitivity in the therapeutic process (Hernandez, 1991; Gaviria and Stern, 1980; Ho, 1987; Dana, 1981; Wright, Saleebey, Watts, and Lecca, 1983; Orque, Bloch, Monrroy, 1983; Gilbert, 1989; Rogler, 1987). However, the combination of older adult status, ethnicity, and caregiving to dementia patients in Hispanic families is a triplet that has only recently received attention (Valle, 1981; 1989; Henderson, 1987; Henderson, 1990a; 1990b; Gutierrez-Mayka and Henderson in press; Henderson, Alexander, and Gutierrez-Mayka, 1989). Unfortunately, the risk of Hispanic older adults entering caregiver roles is sharply escalating due to the expected doubling of Hispanic elders from 4.9% to 9.2% aged 65 and over in the next decades (Hispanic Americans, 1988). This population doubling has serious epidemiologic implications for the Hispanic population due to the association of advancing age to incidence of dementing disease (Henderson, 1990).

The purpose of this paper is to demonstrate the presence and specific nature of ethnocultural themes among Hispanic caregivers to dementia patients so that clinical intervention can be more effective. These findings are part of a larger project designed to test the hypothesis that ethnic minority underuse of Alzheimer's disease support groups on a national basis is a function of sociocultural disincentives and not lack of cases or presence of fully functioning family groups negating need for intervention (Henderson, 1987; 1990b; Henderson and Gutierrez-Mayka, 1989; Gutierrez-Mayka and Henderson in press). This project demonstrated that community health interventions like Alzheimer's disease support groups can be successfully developed in Hispanic populations when ethnocultural factors are adequately identified, understood, and meaningfully integrated into the support group intervention plan. As an analog to this culturally syntonic community health intervention, individual clinicians working with ethnoculturally distinct patients can improve their skills and success by specific inquiry into ethnocultural beliefs and values of their older patients.

The problem for clinicians responsive to ethnocultural factors is how to effectively assess each patient's ethnocultural status relative to their manifest degree of acculturation and their health belief system in relationship to specific complaints or symptoms. The complaint, to be fully comprehended beyond professional practitioner paradigms, must be understood in its sociocultural context (Kleinman, Eisenberg, and Good, 1978; Snider and Stein, 1987; Stein, 1985; Hill, Fortenberry and Stein, 1990; Galazka and Eckert, 1986; Kleinman, 1983; Gilson et al., 1980). Without contextualizing the specific complaints, clinicians are at risk of ignoring or misinterpreting symptoms from an "acultural" perspective, which is by definition limiting and dehumanizing.

The remainder of this article consists of (1) a brief discussion of health belief systems and ethnocultural assessment strategies, and (2) a focus on cases which reveal significant ethnocultural themes among older Hispanic caregivers to Alzheimer's patients.

Health Belief Systems, Aging and Ethnic Minority Culture: Assessment Strategies and Issues

Health belief systems of ethnic minority groups in the United States are usually a syncretism of allopathic, cosmopolitan medicine, and ethnic-specific folk beliefs. Health belief systems include not only etiologic beliefs, but also therapeutic action beliefs influencing health behavior. Also, more general cultural beliefs and values are imbedded in health belief systems and resultant behavior.

Knowing the health beliefs of patients is crucial to effective intervention as a general principle, but is particularly needed with older adults and ethnic minorities. Older adults share several specific life features which make clinical encounters prone to ineffectiveness. For example, cohort effects pertain when the clinician and patient are of different generational groups which are expressed in variant beliefs about gender roles (Garcia, Cuervo, Kosberg, and Henderson, 1989), stigma of mental health crises (Levine and Padilla, 1980; Ho, 1987), greater adherence to traditional ethnic minority cultural values than younger cohorts (Maldonado, 1975; 1985), reluctance to maximally use community helping resources (Cox, 1987; Cox and Monk, 1990; Wood and Parham, 1990), and acceptance of subjugated role behavior in the presence of clinical authority figures (Haug, 1981).

Although usually unacknowledged, cosmopolitan health care practitioners likewise employ health care belief systems. Kuhn (1962) and other historians of science and health care have well demonstrated that clinicians perceive their professionally derived knowledge as "fact" when actually it is an evolving belief system. When a professional belief system is acknowledged, then the structural dynamics of the clinician-patient encounters are more balanced. No one has the edge on possessing the ultimately correct data set. The clinician does not condescend to the patient's "magical" folk beliefs, nor does the patient achieve Enlightenment by elevation to the lofty pinnacle of true clinical fact. Each negotiates an acceptable fit of their health care belief systems to produce more optimal communication, compliance, and treatment outcomes (Kleinman, 1978; 1980; Katon and Kleinman, 1981; Good and Good, 1981; Pfifferling, 1981; Stoeckle and Barsky, 1981; Stein, 1990; Hill, Fortenberry and Stein, 1990).

Clinicians must also make a correct assessment of the patient's location along the "acculturation continuum" (Valle, 1989). On the acculturation continuum, the "traditional position" is characterized by a strong orientation toward their cultural origins and homeland; a "bicultural position" is marked by partial allegiance to their homeland culture and partial affinity with the current mainstream culture; an "assimilated position" is closely integrated with the mainstream culture. Of particular note are the bicultural and assimilated positions because these can be mistakenly ignored by clinicians because they don't appear "ethnic enough" to warrant specific attention. In reality, such people have *not* lost their ethnic minority heritage, they have simply added to it a great facility for using the cultural system of the majority population. Such behavior is in many ways highly adaptive and beneficial. Clinicians must recognize that ethnic minorities who are bicultural or assimilated highly value what they remember as the intent, spirit, or benefit of their more traditional family values and lifestyles. In fact, they may search for "its comforting presence in some surrogate form" (Valle, 1989:129).

Another major aspect of Valle's work underscores the importance of understanding intra-ethnic cultural variation. Valle (1989:131) notes that "culture is not only expressed with considerable variation along a continuum, but also unevenly within distinct domains of daily living where individuals and groups act out their lives. Behavioral and coping responses will situationally change as social environments change. One person's expression of ethnic culture may vary at home, the work place, or the broader community."

Lastly, the stress of caregiving and its episodic crises does not cause caregivers to drop "ethnocultural veils" (Valle, 1989). On the contrary, the ethnocultural response patterns have very often served a positive and protective function in the life of these individuals and families (Simic, 1985). The episodic crisis aspect of caregiving does *not* lessen the presence of differential, ethnocultural response to dementia. Clinicians and researchers alike must be continually alert to the multi-factorial nature of ethnicity in its obvious and subtle expressions.

Determination of case-by-case clinically relevant ethnocultural information is possible using brief interview schedules. These shield the clinician from trait lists purporting to convey the central tendencies of ethnic minority culture and behavior. Strategic questioning of patients can reveal their ethnocultural orientation. However, the quicker the ethnocultural assessment, the more superficial the results. Still, minimal inquiry is better than none. For example, several short interview schedules are available such as the Patient Evaluation Grid (Leigh, Reiser and Feinstein, 1979), the Cultural Health Status Exam (Pfifferling, 1981), the Explanatory Model schedules (Kleinman, 1980; Kleinman, Eisenberg, and Good, 1978; Fowkes, 1988) and the cultural domain matrix (Hill, Fortenberry and Stein, 1990). However, when clinicians are involved in community health programs, more in-depth and comprehensive surveys are required, such as the Snider and Stein (1987) community survey technique and, the most penetrating type, the Ethnic Competence model (Green, 1982; Green and Leigh, 1989). The latter requires a moderate amount of ethnographic data collection, but it is conveniently structured for non-ethnographers to generate a reasonable yield.

SAMPLE AND METHODS

The Hispanic caregivers comprise an opportunistic sample of 37 caregivers and their patients all of whom have some form of dementing disease. These caregivers live in Tampa, Florida and are comprised mainly of Cuban, Spanish, and Puerto Rican Hispanics. The immigration history of Tampa includes an influx of Spanish speaking people from Spain and Cuba in the late 1800's. Many immigrants in this cohort participated in a very large cigar producing industry in Tampa. Later waves of Spanish-speaking immigrants include those related to international politics between Cuba and the USA and a well established migratory path between New York City and Florida among the Puerto Ricans.

The caregivers in this sample were identified from senior adult day care centers, memory disorder clinics, Alzheimer's disease registries, and, very importantly, by a word-of-mouth snowball effect. Data regarding the life experience as a Spanish speaking community member is a product of repetitive ethnographic interviewing of caregivers in their caregiving settings as well as data collected during ethnic-specific Alzheimer's disease support group meetings conducted in Spanish for the Latin population of Tampa. In addition, survey questionnaires were used to record caregiving tasks and frequencies as well as to explicate the Hispanic caregiver helper network configuration.

CASES

The following cases are exemplars in which ethnocultural themes are identified in terms of differential sociocultural response to the noxious behavioral concomitants of dementing disease. Specific reference to Alzheimer's disease is made because most dementias are of the Alzheimer's type and it has become a common, recognized label used informally to mean dementia. In caregiving terms, there is no benefit to identifying a specific diagnosis from the many possible types of dementia because their clinical symptomatology and the resultant caregiving tasks are very similar.

The human expression of discomfort and response to disease pass through unique cultural filters. Home caregivers of Alzheimer's disease patients can be expected to show differences in caregiving styles partly as a function of ethnicity. Such differences can be captured as "cultural themes." Cultural themes are beliefs, behaviors, and/or concepts repetitively used by members of a given social group in the process of adapting to life. Cultural themes may be conscious and explicit in the minds of the user or they may be more latent and detectable only by analytical techniques, such as those found in the Spradley (1979) Ethnographic Interviewing Process or the Green (1982) Ethnic Competence model.

Case #1: Sex-Role Division
of Caregiving Labor and Cohort Effects

The Perez family has had the 68 year-old husband hospitalized at Centro Espanol Hospital with a diagnosis of multi-infarct dementia. The prognosis was not favorable and included complete bed care for the remainder of his life. Consideration of nursing home placement was unthinkable to Mrs. Perez who elected to care for him at their home. The Perez local family consisted of Mrs. Perez' able bodied 88 year-old mother who lived with her daughter and the patient. The Perez adult children consisted of a married son with two small children and a divorced daughter, Juanita, with three older children and one grandchild for which she was providing care.

Having learned at the bedside of her husband's diagnosis and prognosis, Mrs. Perez led her daughter into the hallway of the hospital. Mrs. Perez told Juanita that now it was up to them (meaning she and her daughter) to provide the ultimate in care for Mr. Perez at home. Juanita recoiled and began to list the nearby family members who could likewise lend direct support and assistance but on whom Mrs. Perez was not calling. Mrs. Perez was unable to understand her daughter's reaction in that Juanita was considered the expected helper to the primary caregiver. When a support group for the caregivers of dementia patients was formed at Centro Espanol Hospital, Juanita became actively involved. However, Mrs. Perez was in attendance at only one meeting because of her sense of public humiliation if she had to confront the nature of her husband's disease which produced behavioral aberrations in a public context. Nonetheless, Juanita, who gave occasional "hands on" care, attended the meetings regularly and served as a broker of information and support from the meeting to her mother. The mother was responsive by initiating use of the community services and re-evaluation of her role as caregiver. The patient remained at home with brief episodes of hospitalization for 3 1/2 years before dying at home.

Comment on Case #1

The prominence of the Latin kinship and family dynamic structure is very clear in issues related to burden bearing and responsibility. The foremost of these is the sex biased pattern of familial transmission of responsibility for care of the demented patient. Members commonly report women are expected to provide care for the demented person whether he is the woman's spouse, father, or father-in-law. When the Hispanic family has males and females "available" for providing the major burden bearing responsibility, it is the female who is expected to provide that type of care (Sanchez, 1987). One respondent reported that during the life of the patient (her father), her mother and she would be expected to provide the bed and body care for the patient but that when death occurred, her brothers would take charge because now it entered a business dimension, namely the funeral as a cost item and public display.

Female burden-bearers are virtually a cross-cultural universal (Horowitz, 1985). So what is specifically Hispanic in this case? The answer involves the understanding that ethnocultural traits do not exist as "present" or "absent" bipolar opposites. Such values and ethics have valences and are present in *degrees* and subject to variation based on situation, generation, level of acculturation, intrafamilial dynamics, etc. Also, cultural overlap should be expected, so that the presence of the "female burden-bearer" trait is observable in Anglos, African Americans, Asians, and others. But, the distinctive feature among the Hispanic population is the degree or intensity of expectation which is markedly high.

If the Hispanic family does not have a close, consanguineal female to provide bed and body care for the patient, these duties will typically be assigned to a nearby affine, a daughter-in-law. This provides a source for a variety of intra-familial conflicts. For example, many Hispanic parents are concerned that their adult children may disengage from family responsibilities with the parents. In fact, a daughter-in-law is often the target of great hostility. By marrying the son, she becomes the recipient of attention and help thereby reducing the amount of assistance available to the other family members (del Valle and Usher, 1982). Based on data of Hispanic caregivers to Alzheimer's patients (Henderson and Garcia, 1984), the ranked preference of Latin caregivers by sex and kinship relation in this study is as follows: (1) wife, (2) sister or other adult "blood relative," (3) female non-kin, (4) male "blood relatives," and (5) male in-laws (Henderson and Garcia, 1984). Note that even before switching to kin related male caregivers non-kin females are relied upon.

Clinicians encountering the bias in gender-specific caregiving patterns should be aware of their high intensity of expectation placed on these women in Hispanic cultures. Reticence to change their lot in spite of great complaining can be seen not only as a possible intra-personal psychodynamic feature but inextricably linked to normative values in the network of familial role performance values (Ruiz and Padilla, 1981; Levine and Padilla, 1980; Sena-Rivera, 1980; Canino, 1982; Cox and Monk, 1990).

Moreover, this case shows the effect of cohort or generational variance in adherence to traditional values and behaviors. Mrs. Perez instantly accepted the burden-bearer role but was rebuffed by her adult daughter who expected a more egalitarian division of labor. Ambivalence regarding the discharge of expected roles that the daughter experiences may be wrongly assessed as inter-personal conflict with the parents unless this problem is analyzed in the context of ethnocultural value change across generational cohorts.

Additionally, generational effects are present in the differential response to caregiver support group use. As Maldonado would predict (1985), the younger generation (i.e., Juanita) is more likely to attend and gather information than the older, parental generation. Yet, the older generation will access community resources via the information broker role of the younger cohort. This is exactly what transpired with Juanita and her mother. Clinicians can strategically use this pattern of younger cohort receptivity to benefit an older patient who appears initially to be passive or stymied by the unarticulated array of services and service systems.

Case Example: Stigma

Mr. Garcia has suffered from dementia for several years and is cared for at home. Mrs. Garcia discusses the early stages of her husband's dementia. As she begins to tell of specific circumstances, she begins to explain a Latin ethic. "I tell you one thing about the Spanish, they will get very upset about someone who is crazy or does crazy things." She hastens to add that this is due to lack of education and not just that they happen to be of Spanish descent.

Even during a time when her husband was so confused that he was urinating on the living room floor, Mrs. Garcia tried to direct a facade of household normalcy to her neighbors and even to her children. Mrs. Garcia says "How could I tell my family not to bring a girlfriend or boyfriend here because the house smells of urine." Mrs. Garcia says that even now former friends avoid her due to "fear of the disease" or just feeling uncomfortable about being there. This bothers Mrs. Garcia to the point of wondering if she is being penalized for some past sin.

An event that prompted Mrs. Garcia to put deadbolts without keys on doors of the house involved her husband wandering away from the house at night. She awoke at 5:00 a.m. and discovered that Mr. Garcia was missing. She instantly checked the house to no avail. Her first response was to get in the car alone and scout the neighborhood for him. Only after this proved futile did she return to the house to call neighbors for assistance. They first checked their backyard pool and then decided to drive in separate cars around the neighborhood while Mrs. Garcia waited at home. A neighbor found Mr. Garcia about two miles from home "just in his briefs" with blisters on his bare feet. His safety worried Mrs. Garcia, but the public nature of his "crazy behavior" mortified her.

Comment on Case #2

Alzheimer's disease carries with it symptoms which the general public would interpret as characteristic of someone who is "crazy." The stigma attached to mental disorders is well known within this culture and many others. Escobar and Randolph (1982) report that, for many Hispanics, mental illness is still seen as a dreaded affliction akin to "mal de Sangre" or "bad blood." The issue of a family member being "crazy" has been a common one in the Latin Alzheimer's support group meetings. Members may launch a personal crusade to be sure that friends and family understand that Alzheimer's disease is an organic disease and therefore, not under the control of the individual, thus relieving the patient and family of social stigma liability.

The *concepto de familia* operates to diffuse the stigma of a single case of Alzheimer's disease to all family members. If one has a stigmatized disease (e.g., is "crazy"), the entire family shares responsibility. Public image and respect of others is a crucial value to many. Contaminating this image with deviant behavior, particularly from within a psychotic frame of reference, produces shame and humiliation. However, an organic etiology for this disease releases the family from responsibility and neutralizes the stigma.

The Hispanic caregiver's complex set of reactions to Alzheimer's disease may be submerged beneath a shroud of secrecy or apparent disengagement of concern. Yet, in ethnocultural context, the intensity of perceived stigma is responsible for the caregiver's withdrawn affect, anger or anxiety.

Case Example #3: Cohort/Generational Effects

Maria Lopez attends her first support group meeting in the company of her oldest son. Her stepdaughter had been summoned to go with her, but work schedules prevented the stepdaughter's attendance. During the two-and-one-half-hour meeting, Mrs. Lopez's son, Roberto, introduces her and provides some details of his father's condition. Mrs. Lopez sits quietly during this discourse, which includes commentary and questions from others in the support group, answered by her son. During the support group meeting, Mrs. Lopez herself commented only about her love for Cuban coffee and, due to its strength, the "lift" that it produces from the caffeine.

At the next support group meeting, Mrs. Lopez was again accompanied by her son because the stepdaughter was unable due to work schedules. This time, Roberto Lopez talked mainly about their earlier family life in the Latino quarters of Tampa known as Ybor City. As discussion turned more toward caregiver issues, his mother began to comment in response to her son's status report of her husband's condition. Roberto reported that his father had been very hostile and aggressive for the past few days, to which Mrs. Lopez had responded flatly and quietly, "I'm tired of this. If you don't straighten up, I'm going out this door." Roberto followed her comment by saying that when his mother responds sharply to his father this "brings him back to reality."

Roberto and his mother now alternate commentary about the father's history of being very strict and domineering. Mrs. Lopez summarizes her marriage by saying, "Forty-four years is a hell of a long time."

Eight weeks later Mrs. Lopez is accompanied by her stepdaughter Marcela. Marcela began by saying her stepmother's problem is "lack of sleep." Mrs. Lopez says, "I'm very nervous," and then demonstrates with her hands by shaking them and saying, "Just like this." Mrs. Lopez now becomes outspoken and discusses a history of being physically abused by her husband and occasions of running into the street to solicit help from her other Latin neighbors. In reference to her husband's current condition, Mrs. Lopez is now so bold as to demonstrate his stooped gait and short steps while shuffling his feet. Her stepdaughter interjects that "It's the Haldol" (antipsychotic medication). It is clear that Mrs. Lopez is willing now to express her anger through her raised voice, rapid speech, and physical mimicry of her husband's condition.

Mrs. Lopez refers to her state of "nerves," which is affirmed by Marcela. Mrs. Lopez says that she doesn't take any *medicatinos* for herself because she can't afford them. But she does take honey to ward off heart problems. Mrs. Lopez also says that she keeps her husband fully medicated in order to "keep him cool."

One month later Mrs. Lopez attends the meeting by herself, having been "car pooled" by other members of the group. As a result of encouragement from the group, an aide comes to the home to give Mr. Lopez a bath twice a week. It is now clear that Mrs. Lopez speaks openly and freely within the group setting, having phased herself into the support group family via her younger generation helpers.

Comment on Case #3

David Maldonado (1985) suggests that Hispanic populations variably respond by age cohorts to available helping services such as Alzheimer's family support groups. This age cohort effect has been very clearly observed in the Latin Alzheimer's support group. The most active members are adult daughters and sons of parents who are coping with Alzheimer's disease. The older-generation Hispanics, thus far, seldom attend the group except when specifically brought by their daughters or sons. Furthermore, when knowledge of additional community resources are made known to the parent generation, arrangements for such resources are negotiated through the adult daughters or sons in the group.

It is common to see the older generation Latin person attending the group with an adult daughter or son. The older person sits quietly and occasionally adds an affirmation in response to a monologue delivered by the adult offspring. Usually, however, within a few meetings the older person speaks up, and the role of the adult offspring becomes less important.

Also, it should be noted that Mrs. Lopez more than once referred to her "nerves" and to taking honey to stave off heart problems. This is a manifestation of "nervios." Although usually perceived by professionals in a decontextualized fashion focused on full-blown "ataques" (Mehlman, 1961; Teichner, Caddew, and Berry, 1981; Ruiz, 1982), more recent work argues for a client based analysis (Guarnaccia, DeLaCancela and Carrillo, 1989). In this way, the reality of varied experience and cultural context can be seen. Moreover, even incomplete or partial "ataques" are more clinically meaningful when understood as a variant, normalized, or antecedent version of the complete syndrome (cf. Parades, 1972).

More specifically, Guarnaccia, DeLaCancela, and Carrillo (1989) reinterpret "ataque de nervios" among Latinos as an expression of anger and grief resulting in part from disrupted family organization. Similarly, Low (1981) relates "ataques" to worsening family conflicts. Mrs. Lopez describes some classic symptoms like shaking extremities, and allusion to heart palpitations by her taking honey for her heart. Clinicians are admonished to not over medicalize or psychologize what is essentially a culturally accepted way of expressing psychosocial distress.

SUMMARY

The ability to more specifically determine clinically relevant dimensions of ethnicity by health care practitioners has become more widely available. The increased specificity of ethnic issues for clinicians yields a more detailed and correct cognitive map of client problems and appropriate treatment. Moreover, the individualized approach to patient care is more credible to both clinicians and patients. The net result is that the clinical skill to detect and interpret behavior in the context of ethnocultural systems improves the probability of maximal clinical outcome.

REFERENCES

Busse, E.W. and Pfeiffer, E. (Eds.) (1977). *Behavior and Adaptation in Late Life*. Boston: Little, Brown, and Company.

Canino, G. (1982). "The Hispanic Woman: Sociocultural Influences on Diagnoses and Treatment." In Greenblatt, M. (Ed.), *Mental Health and Hispanic Americans: Clinical Perspectives* (pp. 117-138). New York: Grune & Stratton.

Cox, C. (1987). "Overcoming Access Problems in Ethnic Communities." In Gelfand, D.E. and Barresi, C.M. (Eds.), *Ethnic Dimensions of Aging* (pp. 165-178). New York: Springer.

Cox, C. and Monk, A. (1990). "Minority Caregivers of Dementia Victims: A

Comparison of Black and Hispanic Families." *The Journal of Applied Gerontology, 9,* 340-354.

Dana, Richard (Ed.) (1981). *Human Services for Cultural Minorities.* Baltimore: University Park Press.

del Valle, A.G. and Usher, M. (1982). "Group Therapy with Aged Latino Woman: Pilot Project and Study." *Clinical Gerontologist, 4,* 51-58.

Escobar, J. and Randolph, E. (1982). "The Hispanic and Social Networks." In Becerra, R., Karno, M., and Escobar, J. (Eds.), *Mental Health and Hispanic Americans: Clinical Perspectives* (pp. 122-133). New York: Grune & Stratton.

Fowkes, W. (1988). "Using Patients' Explanatory Models to Negotiate Treatment Simulation with Older Patients." In Llorens, L.A. (Ed.), *Health Care for Ethnic Elders: The Cultural Context* (pp. 33-41), Stanford, California: Stanford Geriatric Education Center.

Galazka, S.S. and Eckert, J.K. (1986). "Clinically Applied Anthropology: Concepts for the Family Physician." *The Journal of Family Practice, 22,* 159-165.

Garcia, J., Cuervo, C., Kosberg, J., and Henderson, J.N. (1989). "Perception of Gender Roles in Older Hispanic Women." Paper presented at the International Congress on Gerontology. Acapulco, Mexico.

Gaviria, M. and Stern, G. (1980). "Problems in Designing and Implementing Culturally Relevant Mental Health Services for Latinos in the U.S. *Social Science and Medicine, 14B,* 65-71.

Gilbert, M.J. (1989). "Cultural Relevance in the Delivery of Human Services." In Keefe, S.E. (Ed.), *Negotiating Ethnicity* (pp. 39-48). Washington, D.C.: National Association for the Practice of Anthropology.

Gilson, B.S., Erickson, D., Chavez, C.T., Bobbitt, R.A., Bergner, M., and Carter, W.B. (1980). "A Chicano Version of the Sickness Impact Profile (SIP)." *Culture, Medicine and Psychiatry, 4,* 137-150.

Good, B.J. and Good, M-J.D. (1981). "The Meaning of Symptoms: A Cultural Hermeneutic Model for Clinical Practice." In Eisenberg, L. and Kleinman, A. (Eds.), *The Relevance of Social Science for Medicine* (pp. 165-196). Boston: Reidel.

Green, J.W. (1982). *Cultural Awareness in the Human Services.* New York: Prentice-Hall.

Green, J.W. and Leigh, J.W. (1989). "Teaching Ethnographic Methods to Social Service Workers." *Practicing Anthropology, 11,* 8-10.

Guarnaccia, P.J., DeLaCancela, V., and Carrillo, E. (1989). "The Multiple Meanings of Ataques de Nervios in the Latino Community." *Medical Anthropology, 11,* 47-62.

Gutierrez-Mayka, M. and Henderson, J.N. (in press). "Social Work for Non-Social Workers: An Example of Unplanned Role Negotiation in a Community Health Intervention Project." *Journal of Gerontological Social Work.*

Haug, M. (Ed.) (1981). *Elderly Patients and Their Doctors.* New York: Springer.

Henderson, A.S. (1990). "Epidemiology of Dementia Disorders." In Wurtman, R.J., Corkin, S., Growdon, J.H., and Ritter-Walker, E. (Eds.), *Alzheimer's Disease* (pp. 15-25). New York: Raven Press.

Henderson, J.N. (1990a). "Alzheimer's Disease in Cultural Context." In Soko-lovsky, J. (Ed.), *The Cultural Context of Aging: Worldwide Perspectives* (pp. 315-330). New York: Bergin and Garvey.

Henderson, J.N. (1990b). "Anthropology, Health and Aging." In Rubinstein, R. (Eds.), *Anthropology and Aging: Comprehensive Reviews* (pp. 39-68). Boston: Kluwer Academic Publishers.

Henderson, J.N. (1987). "Mental Disorders Among the Elderly: Dementia and Its Sociocultural Correlates." In Silverman, P. (Ed.), *The Elderly as Modern Pioneers* (pp. 357-374). Bloomington: Indiana University Press.

Henderson, J.N., Alexander, L.G., and Gutierrez-Mayka, M. (1989). *Minority Alzheimer's Caregivers: Removing Barriers to Community Services*. Tampa: University of South Florida National Resource Center on Alzheimer's Disease at the Suncoast Gerontology Center.

Henderson, J.N. and Garcia, J. (1984). "Ethnic Primary Caregivers to Alzheimer's Patients." Paper presented to the Gerontological Society of America, Chicago, Illinois.

Henderson, J.N. and Gutierrez-Mayka, M. (1989). *Development of Black and Hispanic Alzheimer's Support Groups with Training for Ethnic Volunteer Group Leaders (Final Report)*. Administration on Aging grant 90AM0724, Washington, D.C., 20201.

Hernandez, G.G. (in press). "The Elderly Cubans: Are Their Mental Health Needs Culturally Understood and Appropriately Treated by the Aging and Mental Health Network?" *The Gerontologist*.

Hill, R.F., Fortenberry, J.D., and Stein, H.F. (1990). "Culture in Clinical Medicine." *Southern Medical Journal*, *83*, 1071-1080.

Hispanic Americans (1988). *Statistical Bulletin, October-December*, 2-7.

Ho, M.K. (1987). *Family Therapy with Ethnic Minorities*. Newbury Park: Sage.

Horowitz, A. (1985). "Family Caregiving to the Frail Elderly." In Lawton, M.P. and Maddox, G.L. (Eds.), *Annual Review of Gerontology and Geriatrics* (pp. 194-246). New York: Springer.

Katon, W. and Kleinman, A. (1981). "Doctor-Patient Negotiation and Other Social Science Strategies in Patient Care." In Eisenberg, L. and Kleinman, A. (Eds.), *The Relevance of Social Science for Medicine* (pp. 253-279). Boston: Reidel.

Kleinman, A. (1980). *Patients and Healers in the Context of Culture*. Berkeley: University of California Press.

Kleinman, A. (1983). "The Cultural Meanings of Social Use of Illness." *The Journal of Family Practice*, *16*, 539-545.

Kleinman, A., Eisenberg, L. and Good, B. (1978). "Culture, Illness, and Care: Clinical Lessons from Anthropologic and Cross-Cultural Research." *Annals of Internal Medicine*, *88*, 251-258.

Kuhn, T.S. (1962). *The Structure of Scientific Revolutions*. Chicago: University of Chicago Press.

Leigh, H., Reizer, M. and Feinstein, A.R. (1979). "Approach to Patients: The

Systems-Contextual Framework and the Patient Evaluation Grid." In Leigh, H. and Reizer (Eds.), *The Patient* (pp. 185-195), New York: Plenum.

Levine, E.S. and Padilla, A.M. (1980). *Crossing Cultures in Therapy: Pluralistic Counseling for the Hispanic.* Monterey, California: Brooks/Cole.

Lichtenberg, P.A. and Barth, J.T. (1989). "The Dynamic Process of Caregiving in Elderly Spouses: A Look at Longitudinal Case Reports." *Clinical Gerontologist, 9,* 31-44.

Low, S. (1981). "The Meaning of Nervios." *Culture, Medicine and Psychiatry, 5,* 350-357.

Maldonado, D. (1985). "The Hispanic Elderly: A Socio Historical Framework for Public Policy." *Journal of Applied Gerontology, 4,* 18-27.

Maldonado, D. (1975). "The Chicano Elderly." *Social Work, 20,* 213-216.

Mehlman, R.D. (1961). "The Puerto Rican Syndrome," *American Journal of Psychiatry, 118,* 328-332.

Morycz, R.K. (1985). "Caregiving Strain and the Desire to Institutionalize Family Members with Alzheimer's Disease." *Research on Aging, 7,* 329-361.

Oliver, R. and Bock, F.A. (1985). "Alleviating the Distress of Caregivers of Alzheimer's Disease Patients: A Rational-Emotive Therapy Model." *Clinical Gerontologist, 3,* 17-34.

Orque, M.S., Bloch, B., and Monrroy, L.A. (Eds.) (1983). *Ethnic Nursing Care: A Multicultural Approach.* St. Louis: Mosby.

Parades, J.A. (1972). "A Case Study of 'Normal' Windigo." *Anthropologica, 14,* 97-116.

Pfifferling, J-H. (1981). "A Cultural Prescription for Medicocentrism." In Eisenberg, L. and Kleinman, A. (Eds.), *The Relevance of Social Science for Medicine* (pp. 197-222). Boston: Reidel.

Rogler, L.H., Malgady, R.G., Constantino, G. and Blumenthal, R. (1987). "What Do Culturally Sensitive Mental Health Services Mean?" *American Psychologist, 42,* 565-570.

Ruiz, P. (1982). "The Hispanic Patient: Sociocultural Perspective." In Greenblatt, M. (Ed.), *Mental Health and Hispanic Americans: Clinical Perspectives* (pp. 17-57). New York: Grune & Stratton.

Ruiz, R.A. and Padilla, A.M. (1981). "Counseling Latinos." In Dana, R.H. (Ed.), *Human Services for Cultural Minorities* (pp. 187-206). Baltimore: University Park Press.

Sanchez, C.D. (1987). "Self-Help: Model for Strengthening the Informal Support System of the Hispanic Elderly." In Brown, C.T. (Ed.), *Ethnicity and Gerontological Social Work* (pp. 117-131). New York: The Haworth Press, Inc.

Sena-Rivera, J. (1980). "*La Familia Hispana* as a Natural Support System: Strategies for Prevention in Mental Health." In Valle, R. and W. Vega (Eds.), *Hispanic Natural Support Systems: Mental Health Promotion Perspectives* (pp. 75-81). Sacramento, California: Department of Mental Health.

Silverman, P. (1987). "Family Life." In P. Silverman (Eds.), *The Elderly as Modern Pioneers* (pp. 205-233). Bloomington: University of Indiana Press.

Simic, A. (1985). "Ethnicity as a Resource for the Aged: An Anthropological Perspective." *The Journal of Applied Gerontology, 4,* 65-71.

Snider, G., and Stein, Howard, F. (1987). "An Approach to Community Assessment in Medical Practice." *Family Medicine, 19,* 213-219.

Spradley, J. (1979). *The Ethnographic Interview.* New York: Holt, Rinehart & Winston.

Stein, H.F. (1985). "Therapist and Family Values in Cultural Context." *Counselling Values, 30,* 35-46.

Stein, H.F. (1990). *American Medicine as Culture.* Boulder: Westview Press.

Stoeckle, J.D. and Barsky, A.J. (1981). Attributions: Uses of Social Science Knowledge in the 'Doctoring' of Primary Care." In Eisenberg, L. and Kleinman, A. (Eds.), *The Relevance of Social Science for Medicine* (pp. 223-240). Boston: Reidel.

Teichner, V.J., Caddew, J.J., and Berry, G.W. (1981). "The Puerto Rican Patient." *Journal of the American Academy of Psychoanalysis, 9,* 277-289.

Valle, R. (1981). "National Support Systems, Minority Groups and the Late Life Dementias: Implications for Service Delivery, Research and Policy." In Miller, N. and Cohen, G.D. (Eds.), *Clinical Aspects of Alzheimer's Disease and Senile Dementia* (pp. 277-299). New York: Raven Press.

Valle, R. (1989). "Cultural and Ethnic Issues in Alzheimer's Disease Research." In Light, E. and Lebowitz, B.D. (Eds.), *Alzheimer's Disease Treatment and Family Stress: Directions for Research* (pp. 122-154). Rockville, Maryland: National Institute of Mental Health.

Wood, J.B. and Parham, I.A. (1990). "Coping with Perceived Burden: Ethnic and Cultural Issues in Alzheimer's Family Caregiving." *The Journal of Applied Gerontology, 9,* 325-339.

Wright, Jr., R.W., Saleebey, D., Watts, T.D., Lecca, P.J. (1983). *Transcultural Perspectives in the Human Services.* Springfield: Thomas.

Zarit, S.H. (1980). *Aging and Mental Disorders.* New York: Free Press.

Zarit, S.H. and Zarit, J.M. (1982). "Families Under Stress: Interventions for Caregivers of Senile Dementia Patients." *Psychotherapy: Theory, Research and Practice, 19,* 461-471.

Chapter Five

Pre-Bereavement Factors Related to Adjustment Among Older Anglo and Mexican-American Widows

Bette A. Ide, RN, PhD
Cynthia Tobias, PhD
Margarita Kay, RN, PhD
Jill Guernsey de Zapien, BA

Editor's Introduction

Ide, Tobias, Kay, and Guernsey de Zapien consider the impact of the family system before and after the husband has died: anticipatory grief, widowhood, bereavement, and adjustment. These topics have been covered by articles and clinical comments in previous issues:

Bette A. Ide is Assistant Professor, University of Wyoming, School of Nursing, Box 3065, Laramie, WY 82071. Cynthia Tobias is Director of Medical Computing, College of Medicine, The University of Arizona, Tucson, AZ 85726. Margarita Kay is Professor, College of Nursing, The University of Arizona, Tucson, AZ 85726. Jill Guernsey de Zapien is Program Coordinator, Rural Health Office, Family and Community Medicine, College of Medicine, The University of Arizona, 3131 E. 2nd St., Tucson, AZ 85716.

The original research for this study was supported by a grant from the National Institute on Aging, 1R01 AGO3810-03. A previous version of this paper was presented at the Geriatric Research and Clinical Practice Conference, Orlando, FL, February 16, 1988.

The authors thank Dr. Janice Monk, Research Director for the Southwest Institute for Research on Women, for her advice and assistance with the original project.

1983 I (3) 81-90
1986 V 156, 259, 262, 418, 431, 484
1986 VI (2) 63, 92-93, 140, 142
1988 VII (3/4) 173-176
1990 IX (3,4) 39, 58-59, 74-75, 154, 156, 208
1990 X (2) 73-76

as well as by reviews of selected books:

1984 II (4) 83, 93
1987 VI (3) 82-83
1987 VI (4) 89-90
1987 VII (2) 69
1988 VII (3/4) 90-91

The authors of this chapter discuss a survey which found that, as a group, Mexican-American women tend to be widowed at a younger age compared to their Anglo counterparts. The former are also poorer, less educated, and in worse health. The use of these, and other variables, as predictors of adjustment is discussed with the findings of follow-up interviews and illustrative case studies.

Studies on widowhood tend to disconnect role loss from other aspects of life that may influence adjustment and/or view widowhood from a short-term crisis perspective (Palmore, Cleveland, Nowlin, Raum, & Siegler, 1979; Vachon et al., 1982). This report is directed toward a set of factors that are believed to influence adjustment to widowhood, as reflected in health levels over time. Included among those factors are measures of the character of the widow's relationship with the late husband, a topic that has been addressed by only a few researchers (Hauser, 1983; Osterweis, Soloman, & Green, 1984; Raphael, 1977; Vachon et al., 1982). We pay particular attention to the impact of ethnicity (Anglo American vs. Mexican American) as one of a group of important background factors (age, education, and income level) affecting expectations and subsequent adjustment.

Research on widowhood has neglected ethnic groups other than Anglo or black Americans (Lopata, 1973, 1979). Yet the population of older Mexican-American women is increasing in size and the members are vulnerable to stress due to high rates of widowhood and long-standing socioeconomic deprivation. Between 1970 and 1978 there was a greater increase in the percent of widows among Hispanic women aged 75 and over than among Anglo women in the same age group (Jackson, 1980), reflecting both increasing longevity with better health care and the early deaths of minority males (Cuellar, 1978).

Characteristics of the marital relationships believed to increase the risk of difficulties during widowhood include communication problems (Shanfield, 1979, 1983), high degrees of conflict (Parkes, 1972; Parkes & Weiss, 1983; Shanfield, 1983), and ambivalent feelings (Hauser, 1983; Osterweis et al., 1984; Parkes & Weiss, 1983; Woodfield & Viney, 1984). Such problems may generate later feelings of regret and self-reproach (Parkes & Weiss, 1983) or hostility which is subsequently translated into idealization of the spouse (Woodfield & Viney, 1984).

High degrees of dependence of the wife upon the husband have also been related to poorer adjustment to widowhood (Carey, 1979; Dopson & Harper, 1983; Hauser, 1983; Lopata, 1973, 1975; Parkes and Weiss, 1983). The more pervasive the role of wife and the more dependent the woman on the man, the greater the degree of disorganization and the greater sanctification of the dead husband (Lopata, 1973, 1975).

There are conflicting points of view concerning the role of "anticipatory grief" (Lindemann, 1944) in the grieving process. According to this formulation, when a loved one had died after an extended illness during which there was awareness of impending death, survivors would have time to prepare emotionally for loss in order to mobilize their coping mechanisms (Glick et al., 1974), easing the grieving process and leading to better adjustment. This contention has not been supported by subsequent research (Gerber, Rusalem, Hannon, Battin, & Arkin, 1975; Breckenridge, Gallagher, Thompson, & Peterson, 1986). The usual measure of anticipatory grief has been the length of the final illness, and the survivor's knowledge that the illness is terminal does not necessarily presuppose the existence of anticipatory grief. Forewarning of loss means that one learns to live with the prospect of loss and examines assumptions about one's reality but grief begins with the actual loss (Parkes & Weiss, 1984). An extended illness also allows more opportunity for ambivalence and hostility to develop, the possibility of "waiting vulture" syndrome (Siegel & Weinstein, 1983), the depletion of emotional and financial resources, the gradual social isolation of the caretaker, and physical exhaustion, which can increase the caretaker's vulnerability to illness (Dopson and Harper, 1983; Siegel & Weinstein, 1983; Vachon et al., 1982). In contrast, the occurrence of a sudden death, which allows neither time for good-byes nor preparation for widowhood (Dopson & Harper, 1983; Blau, 1961; Lopata, 1975), has consistently been found to predict a poor outcome (Parkes, 1972; Parkes & Weiss, 1983; Sanders, 1982; Vachon et al., 1982).

Age, education, and economic circumstances have been found to relate to adjustment to widowhood. The widow in the late 50s and early 60s is under particular social and economic stress and has the most problems (Barrett, 1977; Lopata, 1979; Morgan, 1976; Peterson & Briley, 1977; Smith, 1977). Lopata (1973, 1979) has commented that the less educated a woman, the greater is the predominance of the role of mother over that of wife, the more sex-segregated the woman's activities, and the more restricted her social life. Lower levels of education have been consistently related to higher degrees of depression or lower morale (Bahr & Harvey, 1979; Carey, 1979; Ferraro, Mutran, & Barresi, 1984; Kandel, Davies & Ravels, 1985). Lower economic status has been related to anger and guilt shortly after bereavement and poorer adjustment over time in terms of higher degrees of depression and more social and physical problems (Atchley, 1975; Hauser, 1983; Heineman, 1985; Kandel et al., 1985; Parkes, 1972; Parkes & Weiss, 1983).

All of these studies have drawn their conclusions from research on Anglo-American women but research points to the existence of ethnic differences in self-image and self-assessments of both mental and physical health that could affect adjustments. Comparing women of similar ages, Stephens, Oser, & Blau (1980) found Mexican-American women more prone to self-alienation and to seeing themselves as older than Anglo women. Mexican Americans have been found to exhibit lower levels of tranquility than Anglos (Dowd & Bengtson, 1978), higher levels of anxiety (Mirowsky & Ross, 1984), and lower levels of depression (Stephens et al., 1980). Psychological distress has been related to age, the most consistent finding being an age/sex interaction, with older Mexican Americans of lower socioeconomic status having more psychological distress (Burnam, Timbers, & Hough, 1984; Vega, Kolody, Valle, & Hough, 1986). More than one-third of the Mexican-American females studied by Torres-Gil (1978) tended to see their physical health as poor and considered themselves disabled. Comparing older Mexican Americans with Anglos, Blau and colleagues (Blau, Oser, & Stephens, 1979; Stephens et al., 1980) noted that the Mexican Americans tended to be more limited in activity and lower in self-rated health, with the self-rated health of Anglos at age 75 about equivalent to that of Mexican Americans still in middle-age. Nevertheless, some ask whether the differences found between ethnic groups are related to differences in socioeconomic status rather than cultural differences (Becerra, 1988; Kay, 1977).

The classical picture of Mexican-American women describes a traditional view of male dominance in decision-making (Becerra, 1988; Cuellar, 1978; Kay, 1977; Keefe & Casas, 1980; Madsen, 1969; Murillo, 1978; Staples, 1971; Staton, 1972). This was not supported by the work of Cromwell and colleagues (Cromwell & Cromwell, 1978; Cromwell & Ruiz, 1979), who discovered egalitarianism to be the main mode of decision-making across ethnic groups but attitude changes to lag behind behavioral, with the Mexicans believing that husbands should be more influential.

METHOD

The data are from a cross-cultural, longitudinal study of older (40 years of age and older), low-income (under $1000 a month) widows conducted in Tucson, Arizona between April 1984 and September 1986. The study sample included 64 Anglos, 53 Mexican Americans (19 English-speaking and 34 Spanish-speaking), of whom 37.7% were born in Mexico, and six American Indians. This report is limited to the findings from the Anglo and Mexican-American samples.

Three interviews were conducted with the widows at 6-month intervals starting one to six months after the husband died. The interviews contained both open- and closed-ended items. Responses to the former were tape-recorded, transcribed, and later coded using inductively generated categories for quantitative analysis. Consensus among coders was used to resolve uncertainties. The interviews were carried out by middle-aged women, one of whom was bilingual in English and Spanish. Retention rates were excellent; 91% of the Anglos and 94% of the Mexican Americans completed the series of three interviews. The sample of 109 respondents who completed all three interviews was used for the longitudinal analyses. That sample included one black respondent who was included with the Anglo widows because, culturally, her attitudes and ways of life were basically middle-class Anglo (Watson, 1982).

Measures

All measures are based on self-reports and reflect the perceptions of the widow. We measure three aspects of *adjustment*, which refers to self-perceived degree of physical and psychological functioning:
1. *Physical symptom frequency* refers to the frequency of concern with 23 physical symptoms selected and modified from those included in the Project Find Study of the National Council on Aging surveys of 1967 and

1968 (Butler, 1975; Ossofski, 1970). Frequency is measured on a summed 3-point scale of 1 = never to 3 = often.

2. *Psychological symptom frequency* refers to the frequency of concern (measured on the same 3-point scale) with eight items, including "nervousness" from the Project Find symptom list (for which there was consensus among the team members that it constituted a psychological symptom), six items from the Lawton morale scale that have been found to yield consistent results across ethnic groups (Lawton, 1975; Morgan, 1976), and fright ("susto"), a commonly mentioned condition among Mexican Americans.

Internal reliability checks of the Time 1 symptom data yielded alpha coefficients ranging from .78- .80 for the entire scale, .76- .79 for the physical symptoms, and .70- .76 for the psychological symptoms. The psychological symptoms loaded on the first factor to emerge from a Varimax rotation. In addition, a measure of self-rated health correlated significantly with physical symptom level ($r = -.31, p = .002$) and psychological symptom level ($r = -.28, p = .003$).

3. *Functional disability*, defined as a lack of ability to perform selected activities that are generally considered essential components of daily living (Slater, Vukmanovic, Macukanovic, Prvulocic, & Cutler, 1974), is measured by the degree of limitation (none, sometimes, or frequently) in regard to 12 items from the Rand Corporation functional status scales (Stewart, Ware, & Brook, 1977, 1981). It was found to be strongly related to age of the widow and was deleted from the second and third interviews.

Social role independence, or the degree of autonomous functioning in daily activities, is tapped by the wife's *perceived role in decision-making*, developed from answers to one open-ended item: "What did you do when there were important decisions to be made?" Because the only data source was the surviving spouse, this information must be cautiously interpreted (Safilios-Rothschild, 1970). This measure is scaled according to the degree to which the wife had appeared to participate in decision-making: 1 = minimal to 4 = major. A $-.35$ gamma value between this measure and whether the widow saw the late husband as authoritarian lends some credence to its validity.

Dependence is measured as the degree to which activities were shared between husband and wife. The measure was developed from answers to an open-ended item: "Were all of your social and recreational activities together or were some of them apart?" A 3-point scale ranging from low, meaning most activities were separate, to high, or all activities together, is used.

Perceptions of the spouse's qualities is measured in terms of the degree to which he was idealized based on answers to an open-ended item, "How would you describe your husband?" Perceived qualities were categorized as "positive" or "negative," with consensus between coders used where answers were uncertain. The numbers of positive and negative qualities were counted and scaled according to the relative percentages identified on a 5-point scale ranging from all positive to all negative.

Two items measure the *degree to which bereavement was anticipated*:

1. *Length of the husband's illness*, which is measured on a 6-point scale of 1 = less than one day to 6 = more than five years.
2. *Suddenness of death*, which refers to the degree to which the death could have been expected. It is coded as 1 = less than one day of illness and 0 = illness longer than one day.

Social assets are measured in terms of the following: *Age* by age in years, *education* by the highest grade completed in school, ranging from 1 = none to 8 = graduate school, *income* as income per month, coded as 4 = more than \$850 to 1 = less than \$300, and *ethnicity* in terms of self-perceptions of ethnic identity, coded as 1 = Mexican American and 0 = Anglo.

Analysis

The purpose of the analyses was to identify the significant predictors of health levels at each observation time. Stepwise multiple regression, with a .05 level of significance set for inclusion of independent variables, was used for the multivariate analyses. Checks of the distributions of the measures of physical and psychological symptom frequency found them to approximate normal distributions. The data pertaining to functional disability were somewhat skewed so the values were logarithmically transformed prior to analysis. Interpretation centers on the Beta coefficients, which can be interpreted as path coefficients (Blalock, 1972). The independent variables are measured on different units, and the Beta weights make it possible to compare the relative effect of each independent variable on the dependent variable (Kerlinger & Pedhazur, 1973). All regression equations included the following measures as predictors: the sociodemographic measures of age, education, and income level; the measures of idealization, participation in decision-making, and shared activities; length of husband's illness; suddenness of death; and ethnicity. Interaction variables with ethnicity were included in the equations relating to cross-ethnic differences. In addition, each regression equation for the longitudinal analyses included measures of previous levels of symptom frequency, both as controls and because research has found past health level to be one of the most important predictors of present health level.

RESULTS AND DISCUSSION

Description of the Population

Despite their selection on the basis of low income, the two samples differed in various socioeconomic characteristics, living arrangements, and health characteristics (Table 1). The Mexican-American widows tended to be younger and less educated with lower income levels than the Anglo widows. Only three Mexican Americans and one Anglo lived in the

Table 1: Characteristics of the Samples

(Percentages)

	Anglo	Mexican American
Over age 65	52.0	36.0
Less than H.S. education	4.7	86.0
Income < $500/month	31.7	56.0
Live alone	70.3	24.5
Live with children	20.3	67.9
Good adult health quality	71.9	45.3
Greater functional disability	61.0	71.1
Greater physical symptom frequency	67.2	73.5
Greater psychological symptom frequency	64.1	81.2
	———	———
	N=64	N=53

homes of their adult children. The usual pattern of living arrangements was for the Anglo widow to live alone and the Mexican-American widow to have children, adults and/or minors, living in her home (66%). Although the Mexican Americans were younger, they reported poorer adult health and higher frequencies of both physical and psychological symptoms. Many had so little money that they had postponed dealing with their own problems because of the priority of those of the husband.

Results from the Longitudinal Analyses

Our expectation was that levels of adjustment to widowhood would be related to pre-bereavement factors, specifically the widows' social assets, previous health levels, and relationships with the late husband. The results varied with the observation-time after the husband's death. Across all time periods, an additive model best explained adjustment, with no interaction effects found for ethnicity. The significant predictors at each of the observation times are shown in Table 2.

At Time 1 (1-6 months after the death of the husband) social assets were of paramount importance as predictors of adjustment, as reflected in physical and psychological symptomatology. Although the Beta values were in the expected direction for the relationship between ethnicity and the measures of physical and functional problems (Beta = .17; p = .09), no significant ethnic differences were found. Those widows who had lower incomes and were of greater age also had higher levels of functional disability and physical symptom frequency, and low income was the strongest predictor of psychological symptom frequency. Here, lower income levels may be indicative of both past and present stress levels, and the findings support the argument of those who state that ethnic differences may simply involve differences in socioeconomic status. Time 1 then was the period during which the widows, particularly the Anglos, expressed the greatest amount of uncertainty about their financial status.

At Time 2 (7-12 months after the death of the husband), only previous levels of health predicted physical and psychological symptom frequency. Greater age was also marginally significant (Beta = .14, p. = .0515) as a predictor of physical symptom frequency. These findings were consistent with other analyses related to the time of the second interview. By this time, despite the resolution of financial uncertainties by the Anglo widows, perceptions of symptoms still may have reflected the high level of stress present in the daily lives of these widows during this first year of widowhood.

At Time 3 (13-23 months after the death of the husband) greater age and lower past levels of psychological symptomatology were important pre-

Table 2: Significant Predictors of Adjustment

A. Time 1

Health Measure	Significant Predictors	Beta	r^2
Functional disability	Income	-.29	.08
	Age	.27	.07
Physical symptoms	Age	.33	.11
	Income	-.26	.07
Psychological symptoms	Income	-.22	.05

B. Time 2

Health Measure	Significant Predictors	Beta	r^2
Physical symptoms	Physical symptoms-T1	.73	.53
Psychological symptoms	Physical symptoms-T1	.65	.42

C. Time 3

Health Measure	Significant Predictors	Beta	r^2
Physical symptoms	Psychological symptoms-T1	-.27	.05
	Age	.43	.05
	Psychological symptoms-T2	-.27	.06
Psychological symptoms	Psychological symptoms-T2	.55	.30
	Physical symptoms-T2	.30	.03
	Length of illness of husband	.17	.03
	Psychological symptoms-T1	.17	.03

dictors of higher levels of physical symptomatology. The relationship between lower levels of past psychological symptomatology and later physical symptoms was puzzling. Over time, many of the widows had seen the multiple sources of support offered immediately post-bereavement narrow to close family or friends. These findings appear to be congruent with Rosen, Kleinman, and Katon's (1982) suggestion that somatization may provide a way of expressing "troubles" and justifying the need for help, especially for those with more traditional viewpoints such as the older widows in our sample.

Poorer adjustment was somewhat related to specific aspects of the relationships with the late husband. Previous symptomatology together with the length of the husband's illness, with its concomitant strains on the health of the wife and the relationship between husband and wife, were significant predictors of higher levels of Time 3 psychological symptom frequency. The length of the husband's illness was also related to Time 3 physical symptom levels, although not at a statistically significant level (Beta $= .16; p = .08$). The occurrence of a sudden death, which would not have involved the prebereavement strains previously mentioned, was not a significant predictor of adjustment. These results may have been affected by the crudeness of the measure of sudden death (measured in terms of a time span of one day or less); a measure of the widow's perception of the suddenness of the death may yield different results. Also, in this older population, the greater proportion of the deaths of husbands followed long illnesses. The length of the husband's illness had not been significantly related to earlier levels of physical symptomatology, and many of the widows, who had cared for their late husbands for long periods, noted feelings of relief after the death. Supporting the work of those who have commented upon the deleterious impact of an extended illness upon the emotional health of the survivor, the delayed impact of the length of the husband's illness upon psychological symptomatology suggests that underlying feelings of regret, self-reproach, and guilt may have been unresolved.

Two case studies of Mexican-American widows illustrate some of the preceding points, demonstrate generational differences, and show the difficulties in generalizing.

Case #1: C.L. was from the older cohort of Mexican-American widows. During the first interview, which took place during the third month after her husband's death, she was dressed in traditional mourning clothes, and her grandson was present all during the interview. She was 74 years of age and had been married 54 years at the time of her husband's death. She said that her husband had retired in 1975-76 and started getting sick one year later. After a series of operations, he was wheelchair bound with a prosthesis, although death finally occurred from a massive coronary. During the last year, worry and the constant care she took of her husband resulted in difficulty sleeping and weight loss. She was on medication for high blood pressure, heart problems, and arthritis, and reported that her health frequently limited her activities. There was little variation in her psychological symptomology over time, with her scores remaining on the lower end of the continuum. Her financial problems at the time of the first interview were due to delays in social security payments and overcharging at the hospital. She reported her income as being within the $500-850 per month bracket, and she continued the same buying habits as during her marriage, getting money together and paying cash for major purchases.

C.L.'s identified social support system consisted entirely of family—two daughters, one of whom she saw daily and who took care of all her legal/business matters, and a son. At the time of the second interview, a granddaughter and child had moved to Arizona and were living with her. By the third interview, she was ready to ask them to leave, preferring to be alone in her own place. One of her main problems was getting someone reliable to do the yard work. She said that she couldn't rely on the family because they all worked. The only club membership she kept up was the "Club Nacional," a social benefit club to which she and her husband had belonged and where she felt welcome as a single. She said that the club had fund raising events to help people when someone was hurt or died.

Case #2: M.G. is an example of the younger cohort of Mexican-American widows. Born in Mexico, she was 40 years of age at the time of the first interview, which took place about one month after her husband's death. She had lived most of her life in Tucson, and had been married twice; the second marriage had been under 10 years in length. She was left a single parent with four children, two of whom lived at home, when her husband died suddenly from a heart attack at the age of 52 while jogging. Her reported income was also within the $500-850 per month bracket, and she reported problems in obtaining health care, concerns about family members' health, difficulties in making decisions, and feelings of too many responsibilities. Her psychological symptom score was very high at the time of the first interview, moderately high at time 2 and low at time 3.

M.G.'s social support system was not large but did include people outside of family members—a neighbor and a counselor in addition to two sisters. She was open to attending widowhood support groups; she didn't care for Widow to Widow because she saw little in common between herself and the members, many of whom were older and had been widowed 10-15 years. She joined and actively took part in the support group for the Mexican-American widows that was started during the latter part of the project. By the third interview, she had a boyfriend living with her and was thinking of remarriage.

The measures of dependence and independence in conjugal roles and relationships and of idealization of the late husband were not significantly related to adjustment at any of the observation times. The reasons are unclear. It may be that more sensitive measures are needed or that the impact of these factors was limited by the age span and income range of our sample. Also, the generational differences brought out in the case studies may have affected the results. The marital relationships of the older widows would have reflected the more traditional views of those cohorts who married prior to the 1960s, whereas the relationships of the younger cohort tended to be quite different.

Corroborating previous research findings, previous health levels were found to be important predictors of adjustment, particularly during the second part of the first year after husband's death. This finding was one of the strongest and most consistent and has implications for caregivers in regard to early mobilization of resources and support systems. Severe illness and symptomatology were related to prior neglect and inadequate treatment because of financial straits or of priorities widows had had to place upon the health and care of the late husband. The physical health of these low income widows was poor, with a greater prevalence of serious chronic diseases among the Mexican-American widows than among the Anglo widows (Kay et al., 1988). Obtaining health care consumed much of the energy of these widows, who were already depleted by illness. The results suggest that health caregivers need to be aware of the long-term effects upon the emotional health of older widows, no matter what the ethnic group, of strains induced by failing health and a long period of caring for the late spouse.

Particularly important for counselors are the generational differences illustrated by the case studies. Not all Mexican-American or Hispanic women are alike in their views, and age or generational differences may be more important in regard to mental health than the suddenness of the death or the length of the husband's illness. The degree of traditionalism and protectiveness of the family will probably vary with the age of the widow, and younger widows will probably be more open to support groups. The case studies also suggest that the degree of support that can be provided through the traditional close Hispanic support system is being eroded as more women are employed outside the home.

REFERENCES

Atchley, R. C. (1975). Dimensions of widowhood in later life. *The Gerontologist, 15,* 76-178.

Bahr, H. & Harvey, C.D. (1979). Correlates of loneliness among widows bereaved in a mining disaster. *Psychological Reports, 4,* 856-858.

Barrett, C. H. (1977). Women in widowhood. *Signs, 4,* 856-868.

Becerra, R.M. (1988). The Mexican American family. In C.H. Mindel, R.W. Habenstein, R.W. Habenstein, & R. Wright, Jr. (Eds.), *Ethnic families in America: Patterns and variation.* New York: Elsevier.

Blalock, H. M., Jr. (1972). *Social statistics.* New York: McGraw-Hill.

Blau, Z. S. (1961). Structural constraints on friendship in old age. *American Sociological Review, 26,* 429-439.

Blau, Z. S., Oser, G. T., & Stephens, R.T. (1979). Aging, social class, and ethnicity. *Pacific Sociological Review, 22,* 501-525.

Breckenridge, J. H., Gallagher, D., Thompson, L. W., & Peterson, J. (1986). Characteristic depressive symptoms of bereaved elders. *Journal of Gerontology, 41,* 163-168.

Burnam, M. A., Timbers, D. M., & Hough, R. L. (1984). Two measures of psychological distress among Mexican Americans, Mexicans and Anglos. *Journal of Health and Social Behavior, 25,* 24-33.

Butler, R. N. (1975). *Why survive? Being old in America.* New York: Harper & Row.

Carey, R. G. (1979). Weathering widowhood: Problems and adjustment of the widowed during the first year'' *Omega, 10,* 163-178.

Cromwell, V. L., & Cromwell, R. E. (1978). Perceived dominance in decision-making and conflict resolution among Anglo, Black, and Chicano couples. *Journal of Marriage and the Family, 40,* 749-757.

Cromwell, R. E., & Ruiz, R. A. (1979). The myth of macho dominance in decision-making within Mexican and Chicano families. *Hispanic Journal of the Behavioral Sciences, 1,* 358-373.

Cuellar, J. (1978). El Senior Citizens Club: The older Mexican American in the voluntary association. Pp. 207-229 in B. G. Myerhoff and A. Simic (Eds.), *Life's career – aging: Cultural variations on growing old,* Beverly Hills: Sage.

Dopson, C. C., & Harper, (1983). Unresolved grief in the family. *American Family Physician, 27,* 207-211.

Dowd, J. J., & Bengtson, V. L. (1978). Aging in minority populations: An examination of the double jeopardy hypothesis. *Journal of Gerontology, 33,* 427-436.

Ferraro, K. F., Mutran, E., & Barresi, C. M. (1984). Widowhood, health and friendship support in later life. *Journal of Health and Social Behavior, 25,* 245-259.

Gerber, I., Rusalem, R., Hannon, N., Battin, D., & Arkin, A. (1975). Anticipatory grief and aged widows and widowers. *Journal of Gerontology, 30,* 225-229.

Glick, I. O., Weiss, R. S., & Parkes, C. M. (1974). *The first year of bereavement.* New York: Wiley.

Hauser, M. J. (1983). Bereavement outcome for widows. *Journal of Psychosocial Nursing and Mental Health Services, 21,* 22-31.

Heineman, G. D. (1985). Negative outcomes among the elderly: Predictors and profiles. *Research on Aging, 7,* 363-382.

Hough, R. L. (1985). Life events and stress in Mexican-American culture. In W. Vega and M. R. Miranda (Eds.), *Stress and Hispanic mental health, relating research to service delivery.* U.S. Department of HHS, PHS, Alcohol, Drug Abuse, Mental Health Administration. DHHS Pub. No. (ADM) 85-1410.

Jackson, J. J. 1980. *Minorities and Aging.* Belmont: Wadsworth.

Kandel, D. D., M. Davies, and V. H. Ravels. 1985. The Stressfulness of Daily Social Roles for Women: Marital, Occupational and Household Roles. *Journal of Health and Social Behavior* 26: 64-78.

Kay, M. A. (1977). Health and illness in a Mexican American barrio." Pp.99-166 in E. H. Spicer (Ed.), *Ethnic medicine in the Southwest.* Tucson, AZ: University of Arizona Press.

Kay, M. A., Tobias, C., Ide, B., de Zapien, J. G., Monk, J. L., Bluestein, M. & Fernandez, M. D. (1988). The health and symptom care of widows. *Journal of Cross-Cultural Gerontology, 3,* 197-208.

Keefe, S. E., & Casas, J. M. (1980). Mexican Americans and mental health: A selected review and recommendations for mental health service delivery. *American Journal of Community Psychology, 8,* 303-325.

Kerlinger, F. N., & Pedhazur, E. J. (1973). *Multiple regression in behavioral research.* New York: Holt, Rinehart, and Winston.

Lawton, M. P. (1975). The Philadelphia Geriatric Center Morale Scale: A revision. *Journal of Gerontology, 30,* 85-89.

Lindemann, E. (1944). Symptomology and management of acute grief. *American Journal of Psychiatry, 101,* 141-148.

Lopata, H. Z. (1973). *Widowhood in an American city.* Cambridge: Schenkman.

Lopata, H. Z. (1975). On widowhood: grief work and identity reconstruction. *Journal of Geriatric Psychiatry, 8,* 41-55.

Lopata, H. Z. (1979). *Women as widows: Support systems.* New York: Elsevier North Holland.

Madsen, W. (1969). Mexican Americans and Anglo Americans: A comparative study of mental health in Texas. Pp. 217-241 in S. C. Plog and R. B. Edgerton (Eds.), *Changing perspectives in mental illness.* New York: Holt, Rinehart & Winston.

Mirowsky, J., & Ross, C. E. (1984). Mexican culture and Its emotional contradictions. *Journal of Health and Social Behavior, 25,* 2-13.

Morgan, L. A. (1976). A re-examination of widowhood and morale. *Journal of Gerontology, 31*, 687-695.

Murillo, N. (1978). The Mexican American family. Pp. 3-18 in R. A. Martinez (Ed.), *Hispanic culture and health care: Fact, fiction, and folklore*. St. Louis: Mosby.

Nall, F. C., & Speilberg, J. (1978). Social and cultural factors in the responses of Mexican Americans to medical treatment. Pp. 51-64 in R. A. Martinez (Ed.), *Hispanic culture and health care: Fact, fiction, and folklore*. St. Louis: Mosby.

Ossofski, J. (1970). *The golden years . . . a tarnished myth*. New York: National Council on Aging.

Osterweis, M., Soloman, F., & Green, M. (Eds.). (1984). *Bereavement: Reactions, consequences and care*. Washington, D.C.: National Academy Press.

Palmore, E., Cleveland, W. P., Nowlin, J. G., Raum, D., & Siegler, I. C. (1979). Stress and adaptation in later life. *Journal of Gerontology, 34*, 841-851.

Parkes, C. M. (1972). *Bereavement: Studies of grief in adult life*. New York: International Universities Press.

Parkes, C. M., & Weiss, R. S. (1983). *Recovery from bereavement*. New York: Basic Books.Peterson, J. A., & Briley, M. L. (1977). *Widows and widowhood*. New York: Association Press.

Raphael, B. (1977). Preventive intervention with the recently bereaved. *Archives of General Psychiatry, 34*, 1450-1454.

Rosen, G., Kleinman, A. & Katon, W. (1982). Somatization in family practice: A biopsychological approach. *Journal of Family Practice, 14*, 493-502.

Safilios-Rothschild, C. (1970). The study of family power structure: A review 1960-1969. *Journal of Marriage and the Family, 32*, 539-552.

Sanders, C. M. (1982). Effects of sudden vs. chronic illness death on bereavement outcome. *Omega, 13*, 227-241.

Shanfield, S. B. (1979). Social and emotional determinants of the death process. *Arizona Medicine, 36*, 602-604.

Shanfield, S. B. (1983). Predicting bereavement outcome: Marital factors. *Family Systems Medicine, 1*, 40-46.

Siegel, K., & Weinstein, L. (1983). Anticipatory grief reconsidered. *Journal of Psychosocial Oncology, 1*, 61-73.

Slater, S.B., Vukmanovic, C., Macukanovic, P., Prvulocic, T., & Cutler, J. L. (1974). The definition and measurement of disability. *Social Science and Medicine, 8*, 305-308.

Smith, W. J. (1977, May). The etiology of depression in a sample of elderly widows: A research report. Paper presented at the evening meeting of the Boston Society for Gerontologic Psychiatry.

Staples, R. (1971). The Mexican-American family: Its modification over time and space. *Phylon, 32*, 179-192.

Staton, R. D. (1972). A comparison of Mexican and Mexican-American families. *Family Coordinator, 21*, 325-330.

Stephens, R. C., Oser, G. T., & Blau, Z. S. (1980). To be aged, Hispanic, and female. Pp. 249-268 in M. B. Melville (Ed.), *Twice a minority: Mexican-American women*. St. Louis: Mosby.

Stewart, A. L., Ware, Jr., J. E., & Brook, R. H. (1977). *A study of the reliability, validity, and precision of scales to measure chronic functional limitations due to poor health*. Santa Monica, CA: Rand Corporation.

Stewart, A. L., Ware, Jr., J. E., & Brook, R. H. (1981). *Construction and scoring of aggregate functional status indexes (vol. 1)*. Santa Monica, CA: Rand Corporation.

Torres-Gil, F. M. (1978). Age, health, and culture: An examination of health among Spanish-speaking elderly. Pp. 83-102 in M. Montiel (Ed.), *Hispanic Families*. Washington, D.C.: National Coalition of Hispanic Mental Health and Human Service Organizations.

Vachon, M. L. S., Rogers, J., Lyall, W. A., Lancee, W. J., Sheldon, A. R., & Freeman, S. J. (1982). Predictors and correlates of adaptation to conjugal bereavement. *American Journal of Psychiatry*, *39*, 998-1002.

Vega, W. A., Kolody, B., Valle, R., & Hough, R. (1986). Depressive symptoms and their correlates among immigrant Mexican women in the United States. *Social Science and Medicine*, *11*, 35-41.

Watson, W. N. (1982). *Aging and social behavior*. Belmont, CA: Wadsworth.

Woodfield, R. L., & Viney, L. L. (1984). A personal construct approach to the conjugally bereaved woman." *Omega*, *15*, 1-13.

SECTION THREE:
ASSESSMENT OF SPECIAL
PROBLEMS

Chapter Six

Spanish Translation and Validation of a Neuropsychological Battery: Performance of Spanish- and English-Speaking Alzheimer's Disease Patients and Normal Comparison Subjects

I. Maribel Taussig, PhD
Victor W. Henderson, MD
Wendy Mack, PhD

I. Maribel Taussig is affiliated with the Leonard Davis School of Gerontology, University of Southern California. Victor W. Henderson is affiliated with the Departments of Neurology (Division of Cognitive Neuroscience & Aging) and Wendy Mack is affiliated with Preventive Medicine, both at the University of Southern California School of Medicine, Los Angeles, CA.

This paper was presented in part at the 41st annual meeting of the Gerontological Society of America, San Francisco, CA, November 18-22, 1988.

Correspondence should be addressed to Dr. Taussig, Andrus Gerontology Center, University of Southern California, University Park MC 0190, Los Angeles, CA 90089-0191 USA.

The authors are grateful to the following for their back-translation of the clinical and neuropsychological materials: Bill Herrera, PhD, Raquel Camero, PhD, Robert Desdin, PhD, Abel Ossorio, PhD, and Aurea Hernandez, PhD. They thank Oscar Valdez, MD, who was a consultant for the medical terminology, and the staff of the Spanish-speaking Alzheimer's Disease Research Program and the ADRC Clinical Core. The authors are particularly grateful to subjects enrolled in the Spanish-Speaking Alzheimer's Disease Research Program, and the ADRC Consortium of Southern California and to all their families.

This research was supported in part by NIMH (ADAMHA) grant 1R0 MN 43562-01, by NIA grant P50-AG05142, and by the M.R. Bauer Foundation.

95

Editor's Introduction

Taussig, Henderson, and Mack provide an exemplary guide as to how one should go about the process of translating standardized psychometric instruments: Mental Status Questionnaire, Mini Mental, Blessed, Mattis, Boston, Fuld, WAIS, and clock drawings. This careful methodology resulted in translations which passed known-groups validation. Even when variables such as age and education were factored in, there were significant differences between the English and Spanish speaking samples on the Boston Naming Test, Controlled Oral Word Association, Arithmetic Test, and Sticks Test. The other dementia tests (and the Geriatric Depression Scale) showed no significant English/Spanish differences.

The topic of dementia assessment has been one of the most common of all those addressed in previous issues of *Clinical Gerontologist*:

1982 I (1) 11-21, 23-28
1982 I (2) 3-21, 70-71
1983 I (3) 91-92, 92-93
1983 II (2) 13-22
1984 II (4) 3-23
1984 III (2) 23-26, 48-52, 52-54
1985 III (4) 54-57
1985 IV (1) 51-52
1986 IV (3) 3-15, 64, 65, 66-69, 69-72, 84-86
1986 IV (4) 29-35, 40-42
1986 V 19-62, 65, 76-77, 79-80, 84-85, 87
1986 VI (1) 3-14, 59-61
1987 VI (3) 3-10, 59-61, 88
1987 VI (4) 25-34, 35-60
1988 VIII (1) 88-89
1988 VIII (2) 88-89
1988 VIII (3) 27-41
1989 VIII (4) 31-37, 57-60
1989 IX (2) 53-59, 72-74
1990 IX (3,4) 19-46, 67, 68, 72, 73, 114-115
1990 X (1) 29-33, 61-67, 86
1990 X (2) 8-13, 35-66
1991 X (3) 39-45

The number of older Hispanic individuals is expected to quadruple by the year 2000 (Torres-Gil, 1978). As Alzheimer's disease (AD) is the most prevalent dementing illness of old age (Henderson and Finch, 1989), the number of elderly Hispanics with AD can be expected to increase drastically over the next several decades.

Fifty to 70 percent of U.S. Hispanics over age 60 do not speak English (Kemp et al., 1987; Lopez-Aqueres et al., 1984), and it is estimated that up to 90% of older U.S. Hispanics speak Spanish at home (Cubrillo and Prieto, 1987). When a choice of Spanish or English-language testing is offered, respondents who choose Spanish tend to be less educated, foreign born, and older (Roberts, 1981). When assessing these individuals for language, memory and other cognitive impairments, English-speaking professionals often rely on live translators. However, live translators are not only expensive, but they may be unable to convey the nuances of cognition and affect (Sabin, 1985).

There is a great need for Spanish-language instruments designed to assess memory, language, and other cognitive disturbances in AD. However, the development of such a battery would be expensive and time consuming. One alternative is to translate existing English-language neuropsychological materials into Spanish. Such a battery could then be validated in its translated form.

METHODS

Translation

A structured interview, as well as an activities of daily living scale, a memory and behavior checklist, a depression inventory, and the entire neuropsychological battery (Table 1) used with English-speaking older adults enrolled in the Alzheimer's Disease Research Center (ADRC) Consortium of Southern California were translated into Spanish (Taussig, 1987). The translation included the instructions for the clinician, thereby ensuring that the total structured interaction could be in Spanish, and that the original English message would be precisely conveyed. Thus, there would be less possibility that the examiner would use extraneous or inaccurate words that could confound the patient's performance. Careful attention was paid to the fact that certain words in one Spanish-speaking country may be meaningless or offensive in another Spanish-speaking country. The initial translation was back-translated by five psychologists fluent in English and Spanish. They were from Argentina, Colombia,

TABLE 1

Neuropsychological Test Battery

Test	Spanish Version	Reference
Mental Status Questionnaire	Cuestionario de examen mental	Kahn, et al., 1960
Mini-Mental State Examination	Examen de estado mental (mini)	Folstein, et al., 1975
Blessed Dementia Rating Scale	Examen de demencia de Blessed	Blessed, et al., 1968 Fuld, 1978
Mattis Dementia Rating Scale	Escalas de demencia de Mattis	Mattis, 1976
Boston Naming Test	Test de nombres de Boston	Goodglass et al., 1983 Van Gorp, et al., 1986
Face-Hand Test	Test de cara-mano	Kahn and Miller, 1976
Parietal Lobe Battery tasks (Clock, House drawings)	Test de lobulo parietal (reloj, casa)	Goodglass et al., 1983 Henderson, et al.,1989*
WAIS-R: Similarities Digit Span Vocabulary Block Design	WAIS: Analogias Retencion de digitos Vocabulario Dibujos de cubos	Wechsler, 1981 Green and Martinez, 1968
Fuld Object Memory Test	Evaluacion de memoria con objetos de Fuld	Fuld, 1980
Arithmetic	Arimetica	**
Controlled Oral Word Association (F.A.S.)	Asociacion de palabras controladas (F.A.S.)	Benton, et al., 1983
Word list Generation (Animals/ Supermarket items)	Generacion de palabras (Animales/supermercado)	***
Sticks Test	Test de palitos	Butters and Barton, 1970
Trails A & B	Pistas A y B	Bornstein, 1985
Geriatric Depression Inventory	Escala de depresion geriatrica	Yesavage, et al., 1983

* Modification of Henderson et al., (1989) was used.

** The Arithmetic Test consisted of 8 arithmetic problems, one "easy" and one "hard" for addition, subtration, multiplication, and division.

*** Generation of animal names and supermarket items, allowing 60 seconds for each task.

Cuba, Mexico, and Puerto Rico, and all worked without access to English versions.

Back Translation Techniques

Following the approaches of Karno et al. (1983) and Brislin et al. (1973) to back-translation and Brislin's method (1980) for translation in cross-cultural research, the following steps were taken: (1) The original English-language material was translated into Spanish by one bilingual person (IMT). (2) Five bilingual persons without access to the original material back-translated this translation into English. (3) All back-translations were studied to ensure comparability and to reconcile differences among back-translators; by this means a consensus translation was obtained. (4) Finally, a committee consisting of the first author and three of the back-translators reviewed and approved the consensus translation.

English-speaking subjects were administered Similarities, Digit Span, Vocabulary, and Block Design subtests of the revised Wechsler Adult Intelligence Scale (WAIS-R) (Wechsler, 1981), while Spanish-speaking subjects were given the analogous subtests from the standardized Spanish Wechsler Adult Intelligence Scale Escala de Inteligencia Wechsler para Adultos (EIWA) translation of Green and Martinez (1968). Scaled scores were used for both the English WAIS-R and the Spanish WAIS. Therefore, means for each subtest were 10 with a standard deviation of three. This approach was chosen because the Green and Martinez translation is already widely used in Spanish-speaking countries, while the WAIS-R is now most often used for English-speaking persons in this country.

Subjects

Four groups of subjects were studied: 19 Spanish-speaking and 19 English-speaking patients meeting NINCDS-ADRDA criteria for "probable" AD (McKhann et al., 1984), and 18 Spanish-speaking and 18 English-speaking age-equivalent comparison subjects without known neurological disease ("normal controls"). Spanish-speaking subjects were Los Angeles County residents enrolled in the Spanish-Speaking Alzheimer's Disease Research Program. All were monolingual or spoke Spanish as their first and primary language. They were recruited through a variety of community outreach services, including radio, television, and newspaper interviews, in-service lectures to medical and mental health clinics, and educational talks to Spanish-speaking senior citizen centers. English-speaking AD subjects had been previously enrolled in the ADRC at the University of Southern California and were matched for age and for severity to Spanish-speaking subjects on the USC-Activities of Daily Living scale (Hershey et al., 1988). English-speaking normal controls were randomly selected from age-equivalent ADRC normal controls. Informed consent was obtained from all subjects or their caregivers.

For all patients, except as noted below, diagnosis was based on examination findings of a University of Southern California faculty neurologist, appropriate laboratory tests (including CT or MR scan), and screening mental status assessment. For three Spanish-speaking patients unable to see a faculty neurologist, outside medical records were used. All normal controls underwent a brief neurological and neuropsychological screening examination by a neurologist or research nurse. Age of onset was determined retrospectively based on a caregiver's report of initial symptoms. Demographic information is summarized in Table 2.

Data Analysis

Neuropsychological performance was compared among the four subject groups using analysis of covariance procedures. Initial comparisons among the four groups on potentially confounding variables of age at testing and education showed statistically significant group differences on both variables (F(3,70) = 3.57, p = 0.02 and F(3,69) = 8.77, p = 0.0001, respectively). The English-speaking control group had significantly more years of education than both Spanish-speaking groups, and the English-speaking AD group had significantly more education than its Spanish-speaking counterpart. Therefore, to compare test performance between the four subject groups, analysis of covariance procedures were used, adjusting for years of education and age at testing. When a significant overall F-ratio was found for a neuropsychological test, a Scheffe multiple comparison test was performed to determine which groups performed significantly differently from one another.

RESULTS

Mean test performance is presented by group in Table 3. Analyses of covariance showed significant differences in mean performance among the four subject groups on all neuropsychological tests (p < 0.001). There were no differences, however, in scores on the Geriatric Depression Scale. Results of post-hoc multiple comparisons detailing significant between-group differences are presented in Table 4. All neuropsychological tests

TABLE 2

	Group Demographics							
	Sp AD n=19		Sp NC n=18		Eng AD n=19		Eng NC n=18	
	mean	SD	mean	SD	mean	SD	mean	SD
Age at test (yrs)	72.0	9.0	68.2	8.1	76.3	9.8	67.9	8.6
Education (yrs)	7.0	2.6	8.9	5.2	11.1	3.5	13.1	3.3
Age of onset (yrs)	68.5	13.4			70.4	9.2		
Duration of illness (yrs)	4.9	5.0			5.8	2.4		
Severity (%)*	56.4	20.9			58.3	21.1		
Sex (male/female)	7/12		3/15		6/13		9/9	

NC=normal control   AD=Alzheimer's disease
Sp=Spanish-speaking   Eng=English-speaking

* Severity was defined by scores on the USC-Activities of Daily Living scale (Hershey et al., 1988), with decreasing scores (%) representing greater severity

showed significant differences between Spanish-speaking AD patients and normal controls. The majority of tests showed no significant differences between Spanish-speaking and English-speaking counterparts (Table 4). However, there were significant differences in mean performance between Spanish- and English-speaking controls on the Boston Naming Test, Controlled Oral Word Association, the Arithmetic test, and the Sticks test.

DISCUSSION

As predicted, all Spanish-language neuropsychological tests differentiated between elderly comparison subjects and mildly-to-moderately demented AD patients. Although the battery was not designed to differentiate AD from normal subjects, these findings indicate that the tasks are sensitive to the effects of AD. Moreover, on most tasks there were no

TABLE 3

Neuropsychological Test Performance

Test	Sp AD Mean±SD (n)	Sp NC Mean±SD (n)	Eng AD Mean±SD (n)	Eng NC Mean±SD (n)
Mental Status Questionnaire	2.7±2.6 (19)	8.8±1.3 (18)	3.0±2.5 (19)	9.4±0.8 (18)
Mini-Mental State *	12.0±5.8 (19)	28.1±5.1 (18)	12.9±7.8 (19)	29.9±3.1 (18)
Blessed Dementia Rating Scale	13.8±5.9 (19)	32.4±3.6 (18)	11.2±8.6 (18)	25.4±11.5 (18)
Mattis Dementia Rating Scale	73.6±25.6 (17)	130.1±13.0 (18)	94.3±34.4 (12)	147.3±7.1 (16)
Boston Naming	15.6±7.3 (19)	35.9±11.2 (18)	22.4±15.0 (17)	54.6±5.2 (17)
Face-Hand Test	4.8±6.1 (19)	13.0±3.8 (18)	6.7±6.7 (12)	15.8±0.4 (16)

Parietal Lobe	6.8±4.8 (19)	13.6±3.9 (17)	8.4±4.7 (14)	15.5±2.0 (17)
WAIS:				
Similarities	4.1±4.1 (19)	9.6±4.0 (18)	4.1±3.8 (7)	8.4±5.3 (7)
Digit Span #	5.9±3.7 (19)	11.4±3.6 (18)	4.7±2.9 (9)	10.2±3.2 (8)
Vocabulary	6.8±3.2 (17)	10.4±3.0 (18)	6.8±3.3 (5)	10.9±3.5 (7)
Block Design #	3.4±3.1 (17)	6.9±4.1 (18)	3.7±1.4 (6)	8.4±3.0 (8)
Fuld Object Memory	4.4±4.7 (17)	19.1±1.2 (18)	9.9±5.1 (9)	19.2±1.3 (15)
Arithmetic	1.3±1.9 (17)	5.2±2.8 (18)	3.2±2.1 (11)	7.4±0.8 (16)
Controlled Oral Word Association (F.A.S.)	8.2±8.0 (18)	24.5±12.2 (18)	15.9±10.8 (12)	41.5±13.9 (16)

TABLE 3 (continued)

Animals/ Supermarket	12.3±6.6 (18)	35.4±11.4 (18)	13.5±8.5 (12)	41.5±10.9 (16)
Sticks Test	4.7±5.6 (16)	15.9±8.4 (18)	10.3±3.5 (9)	23.4±4.9 (16)
Trails A & B	8.3±12.2 (15)	38.8±15.4 (18)	33.0±11.8 (4)	46.4±9.1 (8)
Geriatric Depression Inventory	9.2±6.6 (17)	8.8±8.7 (18)	11.1±7.3 (11)	8.3±6.5 (16)

NC = normal control   AD = Alzheimer's disease
Sp = Spanish-speaking   Eng = English-speaking

* The serial subtraction task as well as the reverse spelling task were included in scoring. Thus, the total permissible score was 35 rather than 30 points.

Subtests were scored same as the English version

104

TABLE 4

Group Comparisons

Test	Sp AD Eng AD	Sp NC Eng NC	Sp AD Sp NC
Mental Status Questionnaire			*
Mini-Mental State Examination			*
Blessed Dementia Rating Scale			*
Mattis Dementia Rating Scale			*
Boston Naming Test		*	*
Face-Hand Test			*
Parietal Lobe Battery tasks			*
Similarities			*
Digit Span			*
Vocabulary			*
Block Design			*
Fuld Object Memory Test	*		*
Arithmetic		*	*
Controlled Oral Word Association (FAS)		*	*
Animals/Supermarket items			*
Sticks Test		*	*
Trails A & B	*		*
Geriatric Depression Inventory			

NC = normal control   AD = Alzheimer's Disease

Test differences adjusted for age, education

* Statistically significant group differences.

significant differences between performances of English- and Spanish-speaking controls, indicating equivalency of the two versions of the battery.

Significant differences, however, were found on four tasks: the Boston Naming Test, Controlled Oral Word Association, the Arithmetic test, and the Sticks test. Educational attainments were unequal for our two control groups, and for some tasks the English-speaking sample sizes were small;

thus, although we attempted to control for education in the analyses, this variable may nevertheless have confounded our findings. For example, education is known to affect performance on the Boston Naming Test, arithmetic tasks, and controlled oral word association tasks (Borod et al., 1980; Spreen and Benton, 1969). Another issue is cultural relevance. Some of the 60 Boston Naming Test items may be less meaningful to persons raised in a different country or culture. We are in the process of exploring this hypothesis through an analysis of individual Boston Naming Test items. The Spanish-language version of the Controlled Oral Word Association test is problematic for another reason. The relative frequency of words beginning with a given letter of the alphabet is not identical in English and Spanish. Also, in non-Castillian Spanish, the initial "S" sound can be produced by the letters "Z," "S," or "C," and generating words that begin with "S," while suppressing those that begin with "Z" and "C," is a more difficult task in Spanish than English. An analysis of this test by letters (F, A, S) would provide some insight into this problem. With regard to the Stick test, it is unclear why performance of our two control groups differed.

In summary, our findings confirm the utility and validity of using Spanish translations of English-language neuropsychological materials in the assessment of dementia. For most tests in our neuropsychological batteries, English and Spanish versions appear compatible and thus might be used in similar clinical settings.

REFERENCES

Benton, A.L., & Hamsher, K. deS. (1983). *Multilingual Aphasia Examination.* Iowa City: AJA Associates, Inc.

Blessed, G., Tomlison B.E., & Roth M. (1968). The association between quantitative measures of dementia and of senile changes in the cerebral grey matter of elderly subjects. *Br J Psychiatry, 114,* 797-811.

Bornstein, R.A. (1985). Normative data on selected neuropsychological measures from a nonclinical sample. *Journal of Clinical Psychology, 41,* 651-659.

Borod, J.C., Goodglass, H., & Kaplan, E. (1980). Normative data on the Boston Diagnostic Aphasia Examination, Parietal Lobe Battery, and the Boston Naming Test. *Journal of Clinical Neuropsychology, 2,* 209-215.

Brislin, R.W., Lonner, W.J., & Thorndike, R.M. (1973). *Cross-Cultural Research Methods.* New York: John Wiley & Sons Inc.

Brislin, R.W. (1980). Translation and content analysis of oral and written materials, in Triandis, H.C. & Berry, J.W. (Eds.): *Handbook of cross-cultural psychology-methodology.* Boston: Allyn & Bacon Inc.

Butters, N. & Barton, M. (1970). Effects of parietal lobe damage on performance of reversible operative in space. *Neuropsychologia, 8*, 205-214.

Cubrillo, H.L. & Prieto, M.M. (1987). *The Hispanic elderly: A demographic profile*. Washington, D.C.: Policy Analysis Center, Office of La Raza, Advocacy and Legislation, National Council of La Raza.

Folstein, M.F., Folstein, S.E., & McHugh, P.R. (1975). Mini-Mental State: A practical method for grading the cognitive state of patients for clinicians. *Journal of Psychiatric Research, 12*, 189-198.

Fuld, P.A. (1980). Guaranteed stimulus-processing in the evaluation of memory and learning. *Cortex, 16*, 255-271.

Fuld, P.A. (1978). Psychological testing in the differential diagnosis of the dementias. In R. Katzman, R.D. Terry, and K.L. Bick (Eds.), *Alzheimer's disease: Senile dementia and related disorders* (185-193). New York: Raven Press.

Goodglass, H., & Kaplan E. (1983). *The assessment of aphasia and related disorders*, 2nd ed. Philadelphia, Pa.: Lea & Febiger.

Green R.F., & Martinez, J.N. (1968). *Manual para la Escala de Inteligencia Wechsler para Adultos*. New York: The Psychological Corporation.

Hays-Bautista, D.E., Schink, W.O., & Chapa, J. (1988). *The burden of support: Young Latinos in an aging society*. Stanford, California: University Press.

Henderson, V.W., & Finch C.E. (1989). The neurobiology of Alzheimer's disease. *Journal of Neurosurgery, 70*, 335-353.

Henderson, V.W., Mack, W., & Williams, B.W. (1989). Spatial disorientation in Alzheimer's disease. *Archives of Neurology, 76*, 391-393.

Hershey, D.A., Freed, D.M. & Henderson, V.W. (1988). Can brief tests of mental status predict functional behavioral impairment? Presented at the 34th annual meeting of the American Society on Aging, San Diego, California.

Kahn, R.L., Goldfarb, A.L., Pollack, M., & Peck, A. (1960) Brief objective measures for the determination of mental status in the aged. *American Journal of Psychiatry, 117*, 326-328.

Kahn, R.L., & Miller, N.E. (1978) Assessment of altered brain function in the aged. In M. Storandt, I. Siegler, & M. Ellis (Eds.), *The clinical psychology of aging*. New York: Plenum Press.

Kaplan E., Goodglass H., & Weintraub, S. (1983). *Boston Naming Test*. Philadelphia, Pa: Lea & Febiger.

Karno, M., Burnam M.A., Escobar, J.I., Hough, R.L. & Eaton W.W. (1983). Development of the Spanish-language version of the National Institute of Mental Health diagnostic interview schedule. *Archives of General Psychiatry, 40*, 1183-1188.

Katzman, R., & Karasu, T. (1975). Differential diagnosis of dementia. In Fields, W. (Ed.), *Neurological and sensory disorders in the elderly* (pp. 103-134). New York: Stratton Intercontinental Medical Book Corp.

Kemp, B.J., Staples, F., & Lopez-Aqueres, W. (1987). Epidemiology of depression and dysphoria in an elderly Hispanic population: prevalence and correlates. *Journal of the American Geriatric Society, 35*, 920-926.

Lopez-Aquires, J.N., Kemp, B., Plopper, M., Staples, F.R., & Brummel-Smith, K. (1984). Health needs of the Hispanic elderly. *Journal of the American Geriatrics Society, 32*, 191-197.

Mattis, S. (1976). Mental status examination for organic mental syndrome in the elderly patient. In: L. Bellack & T.B. Karasu (Eds.), *Geriatric Psychiatry.* New York: Grune & Stratton.

McKahnn, G., Drachman, D., Folstein, M., Katzman R., Price, D., & Standlan, E.M. (1984). Clinical diagnosis of Alzheimer's disease: Report of the NINCDS-ADRDA Work Group under the auspices of the Department of Health and Human Services Task Force on Alzheimer's Disease. *Neurology, 34*, 939-944.

Roberts, R.E. (1981). Prevalence of depressive symptoms among Mexican Americans. *Journal of Nervous and Mental Disorders, 169*, 213-219.

Sabin, J.E. (1975). Translation despair. *American Journal of Psychiatry, 132*, 197-199.

Spreen, O., & Benton, A.L. (1969). Neurocensory center comprehension examination for aphasia. Victoria, B.C.: Neuropsychological Dept. of Psychology, University of Victoria.

Statistical Abstract of the United States. (1988) (108th Edition) National Data Book and Guide to Sources. (p. 16) U.S. Department of Commerce, Bureau of the Census.

Taussig, I.M. (1987). Taussig Spanish Neuropsychological Battery. Los Angeles, CA: Spanish-Speaking Alzheimer's Disease Research Program, University of Southern California.

Taussig, I.M. (1989). Hearing before the Select Committee on Aging, House of Representatives. In: *Mental Health and the Elderly: Issues in Service Delivery to Asian American, Hispanic, and Blacks* (pp. 22-32). July 8, 1988, Los Angeles, California. U.S. Government Printing Office. Washington, D.C. Comm. Pub. No. 100-694.

Torres-Gil, F.M. (1978). Age, health and culture: An examination of health among Spanish-speaking elderly. In Montiel, M., *Hispanic families: Critical issues for policy and program in human services.* Washington, D.C., National Coalition (COSSMHO).

Van Gorp, W.G., Satz, P., Kiersch, M.E., & Henry, R. (1986). Normative data on the Boston Naming Test for a group of normal older adults. *Journal of Clinical and Experimental Neurology, 8*, 702-705.

Wechsler, D. (1981). *Wechsler Adult Intelligence Scale-Revised.* New York: The Psychological Corporation, Harcourt Brace Jovanovich.

Yesavage, J.A., Brink, Rose, T.L., & Lum, O. (1983). Development and validation of a Geriatric Depression Scale: A preliminary report. *Journal of Psychiatric Research, 17*, 37-49.

Chapter Seven

Acculturation and Depression in Mexican-American Elderly

Kaveh Zamanian
Michael Thackrey
Richard A. Starrett
Lillian G. Brown
Dianne K. Lassman
Annette Blanchard

Editor's Introduction

Zamanian, Thrackrey, Starrett, Brown, Lassman, and Blanchard report on a survey in which both acculturation and depression were measured in Mexican-American elders. The findings were that acculturated and bicultural groups had less depression than the low-acculturation group.

Previous issues of the journal have discussed the assessment of depression:

1982 I (1) 37-43, 97-98
1983 II (2) 3-12
1984 II (3) 60-61
1984 III (2) 28-35, 36, 46-48
1985 III (3) 42-43
1985 III (4) 54-57

Kaveh Zamanian is affiliated with the California School of Professional Psychology, Fresno. Michael Thackrey is affiliated with the California State University, Fresno. Richard A. Starrett, Lillian G. Brown, Dianne K. Lassman, and Annette Blanchard are all with the California School of Professional Psychology, Fresno.

1985 IV (1) 44-45
1986 IV (3) 69-72
1986 IV (4) 21-28
1986 V 97-204
1986 VI (1) 54-56
1987 VI (3) 51-53, 59-61, 65-67
1987 VII (1) 23-31
1987 VII (2) 15-29
1988 VIII (2) 63-83
1989 IX (1) 35
1989 IX (2) 23-35, 37-43, 45-52, 68-71
1990 IX (3,4) 73, 150-152, 159, 174, 184
1990 X (1) 69-73
1990 X (2) 35-66
1991 X (3) 3-13, 73-79, 79-81, 85-87

The purpose of this study is to investigate the relationship of acculturation to depression in Mexican-American elderly. It is argued that this
group's exposure to multiple stressors makes Mexican-Americans particularly vulnerable to depression. First, by virtue of being ethnic minorities,
Mexican-American elderly are subject to lower socioeconomic status, education and language barriers, immigrant status and discrimination on the
part of the dominant society. Second, cultural stressors associated with the
acculturation process create additional psychological distress for them.
Finally, the aging process itself is stressful and is frequently associated
with increased rates of depression.

Depression is one of the most common mental health problems known
today (Wetzel, 1984). While current estimates indicate that 7-15% of the
U.S. population suffers from depression (Chaisson-Stewart, 1985), the
percentage for the elderly is thought to be higher (Blazer & Williams,
1980; Gurland & Cross, 1982; Kennedy, Kelman, Thomas, Wisniewski,
Metz, and Bijur, 1989). A debilitating disorder, depression is more. lethal
in old age (Butler & Lewis, 1982; Klerman, 1983; President's Commission on Mental Health, 1978) because of the alarming rates of suicide
among the elderly.

MEXICAN-AMERICAN ELDERLY

Hispanic-Americans are the second largest minority group in the nation, and Mexican-Americans constitute the largest population within this group (U.S. Bureau of Census, 1984). Mexican-Americans are a heterogeneous group of people who, despite their common ancestry, differ from one another in many respects, such as time and means of settlement in the United States, location of settlement, and diversity of experience (Markides & Mindel, 1987). About half of the elderly Mexican-Americans were born in the United States (Markides & Mindel, 1987) yet have lived in economic and cultural isolation from the American mainstream. Throughout their lives they have held economically marginal jobs and found only rare opportunities for upward economic mobility. Similar to Native-Americans and African-Americans, they have suffered a great deal of discrimination, prejudice and stereotyping (Markides & Mindel, 1987; Roybal, 1988; Varghese & Medinger, 1979).

Elderly Mexican-Americans are vulnerable to mental disorders and are particularly in need of improved mental health services (Markides & Mindel, 1987; Roybal, 1988). Unfortunately, despite the obviousness of their need, elderly Mexican-Americans have received little attention in the psychological literature. The majority of the studies conducted have focused on the general adult portion of Mexican-American population (e.g., Burnam, Hough, Karno, Escobar, and Telles, 1987; Golding & Burnam, 1990; Griffith, 1983; Vega, Kolody, and Valle, 1987; Vega, Warheit, Buhl-Auth, and Meinhardt, 1984). The few studies conducted on the Mexican-American elderly have been narrow in scope (e.g., Cuellar, 1978; Markides, Martin, Sizemore, 1980).

Acculturation

Acculturation is a complex multidimensional process which may occur as a two-level phenomenon, at the societal level (e.g., across generations) and the individual level (e.g., among immigrants through exposure to a new culture) (Berry, 1980; Burnam et al., 1987). Therefore for the purpose of this study, acculturation refers to "psychosocial adaptation to a new culture by individuals who originate from another culture" (Golding & Burnam, 1990, p. 162).

The acculturation process involves conflict as individuals resolve cultural differences with the new environment. This conflict, termed "acculturative stress" (Berry, 1980; Born, 1970, cited in Mena, Padilla, and Maldonado, 1987, p. 208), is often associated with various psychological consequences such as depression (Burnam et al., 1987; Golding & Burnam, 1990; Griffith, 1983). A review of the literature clearly reveals that differences in level of acculturation play a crucial role in an individual's psychological well-being (Burnam et al., 1987; Griffith, 1983; Ortiz & Arce, 1984; Szapocznik & Kurtines, 1980).

With respect to Mexican-Americans, various positions have been taken regarding the relationship between acculturation and mental disorders. A review of the literature reveals three conflicting hypotheses about this relationship. First, some authors have proposed that higher rates of psychological distress are evident among the less acculturated individuals. The psychological effects of acculturation, similar to effects of a crisis situation, are regarded as psychologically stressful to the individual. It is postulated that as a result of contact with a new cultural system, an individual's life undergoes a substantial degree of change, to the extent that it may challenge the person's ability to cope with the psychological demands of adaptation (Fabrega, 1969). This hypothesis views acculturation as a challenge to the personal belief systems, customs, and values of an individual. From this perspective acculturation involves a degree of social change which undermines traditional values, security and stability of the family system, leading to disruptions of customary life patterns which in turn lead to psychological distress. This position has been supported by various investigators (Fabrega and Wallace, 1970; Vega, Warheit, and Meinhardt, 1984).

Other authors have argued that less acculturated individuals are at lower risk for experiencing psychological distress. This position is based on the assumption that retention of customs and values of the mother culture is "healthier" than its abandonment. In respect to Mexican-Americans, it has been suggested that the strong family orientation and social ethics of the Mexican culture result in less distress among the unacculturated than among those who have abandoned these resources by acculturating to "Anglo" norms (Graves, 1967; Madsen, 1964). The authors propose that acculturation leads to alienation and isolation from the supportive Mexican-American community while efforts to achieve status in a discriminatory Anglo society are frustrated. Madsen (1964) notes that Mexican-Americans attempting to acculturate to the dominant culture are "trapped" in a stressful and anxiety provoking situation which will result in higher rates of psychopathology.

The third and most recent perspective on the relationship between acculturation and psychological distress is the bicultural hypothesis. The bicultural view proposes that individuals who have integrated and adapted the values and behaviors of two or more cultures are less likely to experience psychological distress than are monocultural persons (Buriel, 1984; Ramirez, 1984; Szapocznik & Kurtines, 1980). This position maintains that monocultural individuals are less likely to be flexible in coping with or adapting to the bicultural or multicultural milieu of the overall society, and are therefore more likely to experience psychological distress (Szapocznik & Kurtines, 1980). Several investigators have argued that bicultural or multicultural individuals as a result of their expanded skills and knowledge of the different cultures, are more flexible, adaptable, and better equipped for today's pluralistic society (McFee, 1968; Ramirez, 1969; 1984; Szapocznik, 1980). None of the hypotheses noted is particularly well supported; the need for further investigation is evident.

METHOD

Design and Sample

The data were obtained from telephone interviews conducted in Fresno, California with 159 Mexican-American subjects 60 years of age and over. The respondents were identified by a listing of Spanish-surnames provided by the United States Immigration and Naturalization services, and were randomly selected using the Polk telephone directory that lists the names of residents of the city of Fresno by the prefix of their telephone numbers. The sampling error was estimated at 5%. College educated, bilingual interviewers conducted the telephone surveys.

Measures

The questionnaire used for this study was part of a larger research project. For the purposes of the current project, several assessment devices were used to obtain the following categories of information: screening and introduction; demographic/socioeconomic information; depression inventories; and acculturation. Each participant responded to Hollingshead's Four Factor Index (Hollingshead, 1975), the Geriatric Depression Scale (GDS) (Brink, Yesavage, Lum, Heeresema, Adey, & Rose, 1982; see Appendix III), the Center for Epidemiological Studies Depression Scale (CES-D) (Radloff, 1977), and the Acculturation Rating Scale for Mexican-Americans (ARSMA) (Cuellar, Harris, & Jasso, 1980).

The screening and introduction section served several purposes. As a screening procedure it was used to determine whether persons contacted were part of the population under investigation (i.e., Mexican-American 60 years or older). If qualified, the persons contacted were informed of the project's purpose and aim, and were advised of the confidential nature of the investigation. Upon the respondent's consent the interviewers proceeded with the interview. Demographic information was obtained and socioeconomic status was established by combining information on sex, marital status, education, and occupation on Hollingshead's Four Factor Index (Hollingshead, 1975). Level of depression was assessed using the Geriatric Depression Scale (GDS) and the Center for Epidemiologic Studies Depression Scale (CES-D).

The CES-D was specifically devised to estimate the prevalence of depressive symptomatology in the general population (Radloff, 1977). This self-report instrument consists of 20 items selected from a larger pool of items used in previously validated measures of depression. The CES-D items cover cognitive, affective, behavioral, and somatic symptoms associated with depression. For each item, respondents indicate the frequency or duration with which a specific depressive feature has occurred during the preceding week. Respondents describe their mood by rating each item as 0 = rarely or none of the time, 1 = some or a little of the time, 2 = occasionally or a moderate amount of time, or 3 = more or all of the time. Total scores, calculated by summing responses to all 20 items, can range from 0 to 60, with higher scores indicating greater distress. A number of factor analytic, reliability and validity studies have confirmed the scale's psychometric properties (Aneshensel, Clark, and Frerichs, 1983; Clark, Aneshensel, Frerichs, and Morgan, 1981; Devins, Orme, Costello, Binik, Frizzell, Stam, and Pullin, 1988; Golding and Aneshensel, 1989; Roberts, 1980; and Weissman, Sholomskas, Pottenger, Prusoff, and Locke, 1977). Recently the CES-D has been widely used with the Mexican-American population (Garcia & Marks, 1988; Golding & Burnam, 1990; Golding and Karno, 1988; Markides & Krause, 1981; Markides & Vernon, 1984; Vega and Kolody, 1987; and Vega, Kolody, Valle, 1986), and its psychometric properties prevailed despite the cultural differences (Aneshensel, Clark, and Frerichs, 1983; Clark, Aneshensel, Frerichs, and Morgan, 1981; Golding and Aneshensel, 1989).

The Geriatric Depression Scale (GDS) (Brink et al., 1982) (see Appendix III) was devised in response to the absence of a depression inventory specifically tailored for the elderly. The GDS is a brief self-report instrument which is less sensitive than other depression inventories to depressive features of old age that are often confounded with the normal aging process (Hyer and Blount, 1984). This 30-item inventory moves away from questions that are heavily loaded toward vegetative symptoms, therefore does not emphasize such variables as physical complains, reduced libido, and appetite problems. Each item is answered in a true/false format which fosters easy administration especially for debilitated elderly. The scale's reliability and validity have been demonstrated with community residents as well as with those under medical or psychiatric care in inpatient and outpatient settings Koenig, Meador, Cohen, and Blazer, 1988; Norris, Gallagher, Wilson, and Winogard, 1987; Parmelee, Lawtin, Katz, 1989; and Yesavage, Brink, Lum, Huang, Adey, and Leirer, (1983).

The Acculturation Rating Scale for Mexican-Americans (ARSMA) consists of 20 questions each scored on a five-point Likert scale ranging from Mexican/Spanish to Anglo/English. The scale covers dimensions of language familiarity and usage, ethnic interaction, ethnic pride and identity, cultural heritage, and generational proximity. The ARSMA is available in both Spanish and English and may be administered individually, as a group test, or as a self-report measure. Reliability and validity of ARSMA have been demonstrated by the original authors (Cuellar, Harris, and Jasso, 1980) and other investigators (Montgomery and Orozco, 1984). A number of authors have utilized ARSMA or modified versions of it as an acculturation measure (Alatorre-Alva, 1985; Burnam, Telles, Hough, and Escobar, 1987; Domino & Acosta, 1987; Ghaffarian, 1987; Golding & Burnam, 1990; and Vega, Kolody, & Valle, 1988). Typically ARSMA is scored by dividing the total score by the number of items answered. This procedure produces a score in the range from 1 "very Mexican" to 5 "very Anglicized." These continuous scores are categorized into five "types" of acculturation (Cuellar et al., 1980): (1) very Mexican, scores of 1.00 to 1.99; (2) Mexican-oriented bicultural, scores of 2.00 to 2.79; (3) true bicultural, scores of 2.80 to 3.20; (4) Anglo-oriented bicultural, scores of 3.21 to 4.00; (5) very Anglicized, scores of 4.01 to 5.00. For the purpose of this study, a respondent's total acculturation score (in the range from 0 to 100) places him or her into one of three groups. The groups were determined based on a frequency distribution of the overall number of respondents who completed the scale. The individuals with an overall acculturation score of 0 to 39 are considered to be in the low acculturated group, scores of 40 to 57 are bicultural, and scores of 57 to 100 constitute high acculturation.

RESULTS

Depression scores on both the GDS and the CES-D were clearly associated with acculturation: Low acculturated persons scored consistently higher than either highly acculturated or bicultural persons. This relationship, evaluated with separate one way ANOVAs for the GDS and the CES-D measures respectively, was significant in both cases (GDS F2, 156 = 11.85; $p < .001$; CES-D F2,151 = 11.04; $p < .001$). Mean scores for the low-acculturated, bicultural, and high-acculturated groups on the GDS and CES-D were 9.92, 5.84, and 4.47 and 14.46, 7.46, and 5.62, respectively. The data did not support the "bicultural hypothesis"; in fact the middle (bicultural) group showed a striking resemblance to the high-acculturated group. Both the bicultural and high-acculturated groups showed lower signs of depression than did the low-acculturated group. Socioeconomic status (SES) did not mitigate the observed relationship of acculturation to depression, as the SES covariate had no effect on either GDS (F1,150 = 1.52; p = .22) or CES-D (F1,150 = 1.29; p = .26).

DISCUSSION

A clear inverse relationship between acculturation and depression was obtained. Participants in this study who were minimally acculturated to the United States responded to both depression measures with more evidence of distress than either highly acculturated or bicultural individuals, whose scores were quite similar.

This suggests that although elderly persons who are bicultural are less likely to be depressed than are elderly monocultural Mexican persons, the biculturality in and of itself is not preferable to being monocultural Anglo. In fact, our results imply that letting go of the Mexican culture in favor of the dominant (Anglo) culture may buffer one against depression. Contrary to the assumptions of the bicultural hypothesis, abandoning the Mexican culture does not result in increased distress, and instead, incorporating aspects of the dominant culture is associated with lower levels of depression.

The strong relationship between low acculturation and high depression scores in Mexican-American elderly indicates that retention of aspects of Mexican culture without concomitant attempts to incorporate aspects of the dominant culture results in the most vulnerable position to depression. This is very probably attributable to social isolation of low acculturated Mexican-American elderly, whose lack of familiarity or comfort with dominant culture activities or norms may keep them from venturing out to seek and establish social networks. Church and extended family, two groups known to buffer against distress and to be associated with psychological well being in Mexican-Americans may be less accessible to this group of under-acculturated persons.

In view of the absence of socioeconomic status as a mitigating factor, it is imperative to note that several variables such as health, income, and poor housing are not addressed in this study. These factors constitute additional sources of distress for the aged Mexican-Americans, contributing to their susceptibility to mental health problems in general and depression in particular.

Levels of acculturation and degree of familiarity with the host culture are viable factors to consider in individual and family therapy with Mexican-American elderly persons. Efforts should be made to encourage low acculturated individuals to increase their familiarity with the mainstream culture. Socialization and structured activity programs emphasizing elements of both the Anglo and Mexican cultures might be particularly well suited for low acculturated elderly persons.

REFERENCES

Alatorre-Alva, S. (1985). The political acculturation of Mexican-American adolescents. *Hispanic Journal of Behavioral Sciences*, Vol 7(4), 345-364.

Aneshensel, C.S., Clark, V.A., and Frerichs, R.R. (1983). Race, ethnicity, and depression: A confirmatory analysis. *Journal of Personality and Social Psychology*, Col 44, 385-398.

Berry, J. W., (1980). Acculturation as varieties of adaptation. In A. Padilla (Ed.), Acculturation: Theory models and some new findings. Boulder: Westview.

Blazer, D., Williams, C.D. (1980). Epidemiology of dysphoria and depression in an elderly population. *American Journal of Psychiatry*, Vol 134(4), 439-444.

Burvill, P.W., Hall, W.D., Stampfer, H.G., and Emmerson, J.P. (1989). A comparison of early-onset and late-onset depressive illness in the elderly. *American Journal of Psychiatry*, Vol 155, 673-679.

Brink, T.L., Yeavage, J., Lum, O., Heeresema, P.H., Adey, M., & Rose, T.L. (1982). Screening tests for geriatric depression. *Clinical Gerontology*, 10, 37-44.

Buriel, R. (1984). Integration with traditional Mexican-American culture and sociocultural adjustment. *Chicano Psychology*, 2nd edition, New York: Academic Press.

Burnam, M.A., Hough, R.L., Karno, M., Escobar, J.I., Telles, C.A., (1987). Acculturation and lifetime prevalence of psychiatric disorders among Mexican Americans in Los Angeles. *Journal of Health and Social Behavior,* 28(Mar), 89-102.

Burnam, M.A., Telles, C.A., Hough, R.L., Escobar, J.L. (1987). Measurement of acculturation in a community population of Mexican Americans. *Hispanic Journal of Behavioral Sciences,* 9(2), 105-130.

Butler, R.N., & Lewis, M.I. (1982). *Aging and Mental Health: Positive Psychosocial Approaches*, Saint Louis: The C.V. Mosby Company.

Califano, J.A. (1978). The aging America: Questions for the four-generation society. *The Annals of the American Academy*, 438, 96-107.

Chaisson-Stewart, M.G. (1985). Depression incidence: Past, present, and future. *Depression in the Elderly: An Interdisciplinary Approach*. A Wiley Medical Publication: John Wiley & Sons.

Clark, V.A., Aneshensel, C.S., Frerichs, R.R., Morgan, T.M. (1981). Analysis of effects of sex and age in response to items on the CES-D scale. *Psychiatry Research*, Vol 5, 171-181.

Cuellar, J.B. (1978). El Senior citizens club: The older Mexican-American in the voluntary association. *Life's Career-Aging: Cultural Variations on Growing Old*, 1st Edition. Beverly Hills: Sage Publications, Inc.

Cuellar, I., Harris, L.C., & Jasso, R. (1980). An acculturation scale for Mexican American normal and clinical populations. *Hispanic Journal of Behavioral Sciences, 3*, 199-217.

Devins, G.M., Orme, C.M., Costello, C.G., Binik, Y.M., Frizzell, B., Stam, H.J., Pullin, W.M. (1988). Measuring depressive symptoms in illness populations: Psychometric properties of the Center for Epidemiologic Studies Depression (CES-D) Scale. *Psychology and Health*, vol 2, 139-156.

Domino, G., & Acosta, A. (1987). The relation of acculturation and values in Mexican-Americans. *Hispanic Journal of Behavioral Sciences*, Vol 9(2), 131-150.

Fabrega, H. (1969). Social psychiatric aspects of acculturation and migration: A general statement. *Comprehensive Psychiatry*, 10, 314-326.

Fabrega, H., Wallace, C. A. (1970). Acculturation and psychiatric treatment: A study involving Mexican-Americans. *British Journal of Social Psychiatry and Community Health*, 4, 124-136.

Garcia, M. & Marks, G. (1988). Depressive symptomatology among Mexican-American adults: An examination with the CES-D scale. *Psychiatry Research*, Vol 27, 137-148.

Ghaffarian, S. The Acculturation of Iranians in the United States. *Journal of Social Psychology, 127*(6), 565-571.

Golding, J.M., Aneshensel, C.S. (1989). Factor structure of the Center for Epidemiologic Studies Depression Scale among Mexican-Americans and non-Hispanic Whites. *Psychological Assessment*, Vol 1(3), 163-168.

Golding, J.M., Burnam, M.A. (1990). Immigration, stress, and depressive symptoms in a Mexican-American community. *Journal of Nervous and Mental Disease*, 178(3), 161-171.

Golding J.M., Karno, M. (1988). Gender differences in depressive symptoms among Mexican-Americans and Non-Hispanic whites. *Hispanic Journal of Behavioral Sciences*, 10(1), 1-19.

Graves, T.D. (1967). Acculturation, access and alcohol in a tri-ethnic community. *American Anthropologist, 69*, 306-321.

Griffith, J. (1983). Relationship between acculturation and psychological impairment in adult Mexican Americans. *Hispanic Journal of Behavioral Science, 5*, 431-459.

Gurland, B.J., & Cross, P.S. (1982). Epidemiology of psychopathology in old age. *Psychiatric Clinics of North America*, Vol 5(1), 11-25.

Hale, W.D., Cochran, C.D. (1986). Gender differences in health attitudes among the elderly. *Clinical Gerontologist*, 4(3), 23-27.

Hill, R.D., Gallagher, D., Thompson, L.W., Ishida, T. (1988). Hopelessness as a measure of suicidal intent in the depressed elderly. *Psychology and Aging*, Vol 3(3), 230-232.

Hollingshead, A.B. (1975). Four-factor index of social status. New Haven: Yale University.

Hyer, L. & Blount, J. (1984). Concurrent and discriminant validities of the Geriatric Depression Scale with older psychiatric inpatients. *Psychological Reports*, Vol 54, 611-616.

Kennedy, G.J., Kelman, H.R., Thomas, C., Wisniewski, W., Metz, H., and Bijur, P.E. (1989). Hierarchy of characteristics associated with depressive symptoms in an urban sample. *American Journal of Psychiatry*, 146:2, February.

Koenig, H.G., Meador, K.G., Cohen, H.J., & Blazer, D.G. (1988). Self-rated depression scales and screening for major depression in the older hospitalized patient with medical illness. *Journal of the American Geriatric Society*, Vol 36, 699-706.

Larson, R. (1978). Thirty years of research on the subjective well-being of older Americans. *Journal of gerontology*, 33(1), 109-125.

Lasoski, M.C., Thelen, M.H. (1987). Attitudes of older and middle-aged persons toward mental health intervention. *The Gerontological Society of America*, 27(3), 288-292.

Madsen, W. (1964). The alcoholic agringado. *American Anthropologist*, 66, 355-361.

Markides, K.S., & Kraus, N. (1985). Intergenerational solidarity and psychological well-being among older Mexican-Americans: A three generations study. *Journal of Gerontology*, Vol 40, 390-392.

Markides, K.S., & Martin, H.W., and Sizemore, M. (1980). Psychological distress among elderly Mexican-Americans and Anglos. *Ethnicity*, Vol 7, 298-309.

Markides, K.S., & Mindel, C.H. (1987). *Aging & Ethnicity*. Beverly Hills: Sage Publications.

Markides, K.S., Vernon, S. (1984). Aging, sex-role orientation, and adjustment: A three generations study of Mexican-Americans. *Journal of Gerontology*, Vol 39, 586-591.

McFee, M. (1968). The 150% man: A product of blackfeet acculturation. *American Anthropologist*, Vol 70, 1096-1107.

Mena, F., Padilla, A.M., Maldonado, M. (1987). Acculturative stress and specific coping strategies among immigrant and later generation college students. *Hispanic Journal of Behavioral Sciences*, 9(2), 207-225.

Milazzo, L.J., Benson, P.R., Rosenstein, M.J., Manderscheld, R.W. (1987).

Use of inpatient psychiatric services by the elderly age 65 and over, United States, 1980. Statistical Note.

Montgomery, G.T., & Orozco, S. (1984). Validation of a measure of acculturation for Mexican-Americans. *Hispanic Journal of Behavioral Sciences*, Vol 6, 53-63.

Norris, J.T,. Gallagher, D., Wilson, A., & Winogard, C.H. (1987). Assessment of depression in geriatric medical outpatients: The validity of two screening measures. *Journal of the American Geriatric Society*, Vol 35, 989-995.

Ortiz, V., Acre, C.H. (1984). Language orientation and mental health status among persons of Mexican descent. *Hispanic Journal of Behavioral Sciences*, 6, 127-143.

Parmelee, P.A., Lawton, M.P., and Katz, I.R. (1989). Psychometric properties of the Geriatric Depression Scale among the institutionalized aged. *Psychological Assessment*, Vol 1(4), 331-338.

President's Commission on mental health, Report of the special populations panel on mental health of Mexican-Americans. Submitted to The President's Commission on Mental Health, February, 15, 1978.

Radloff, L.S. (1977). The CES-D scale: A self-report depression scale for research in the general population. *Applied Psychological Measurement*, 1(3), 385-401.

Ramirez, M. (1969). Identification with Mexican-American values and psychological adjustment in Mexican-American adolescents. *International Journal of Social Psychiatry*, Vol 15, 151-156.

Ramirez, M. (1984). Assessing and understanding Biculturalism-Multiculturalism in Mexican American adults. *Chicano Psychology*, 2nd Edition, New York: Academic Press.

Redfield, R., Linton, R., & Herskovitz, M.J. (1936). Memorandum on the study of acculturation. *American Anthropologist*, Vol 38, 149-152.

Roberts, R.E. (1980). Reliability of the CES-D scale in different ethnic contexts. *Psychiatry Research*, Vol 2, 125-134.

Rosenwaike, I. (1985). A demographic portrait of the oldest old. *Health and Society*, 63(2), 187-205.

Roybal, E.R. (1988). Mental health and aging. *American Psychologist*, Vol 43(3), 189-194.

Schonfeld, L., Garcia, J., Streuber, P. (1985). Factors contributing to mental health treatment of the elderly. *Journal of Applied Gerontology*, 4(2), 30-39.

Szapocznik, J. & Kurtines, W. (1980). Acculturation, biculturalism, and adjustment among Cuban Americans. In A. Padilla (Ed.), Acculturation: Theory, models and some new findings. Boulder: Westview.

Templer, D.I., & Cappalletty, G.G. (1986). Suicide in the elderly: Assessment and intervention. In T.L. Brink (Ed.), *Clinical Gerontology: A guide to assessment and intervention* (pp 475-487). New York: Hawthorn Press.

U.S. Bureau of the Census. Persons of Spanish Origin in the United States: March 1980 (Advance report). Series P-20, No 361, Issued May 1981.

Varghese, R., & Medinger, F. (1979). Fatalism in response to stress among the minority aged. *Ethnicity and Aging: Theory, research, and policy*, New York: Springer Publishing Company.

Vega, W.A., Kolody, B., Valle, R. (1988). Marital strain, coping, and depression among Mexican-American women. *Journal of Marriage and the Family*, 50, 391-403.

Vega, W.A., Kolody, B., Valle, R. (1987). Migration and mental health: An Empirical test of depression risk factors among immigrant Mexican women. *Migration and Health*, 21(3), 512-529.

Vega, W.A., Kolody, B., Valle, R. (1986). The relationship of marital status, confident support, and depression among Mexican immigrant women. *Journal of Marriage and the Family*, 48, 597-605.

Vega, W.A., Warheit, G. Buhl-Auth, J., and Meinhardt, K. (1984). The prevalence of depressive symptoms among Mexican-Americans and Anglos. *American Journal of Epidemiology*, Vol 120, 592-607.

Vega, W.A., Warheit, G., Meinhardt, K. (1984). Marital disruption and the prevalence of depressive symptomatology among Anglos and Mexican Americans. *Journal of Marriage and Family*, 4, 817-824.

Weinberger, M., Darnell, J.C., Martz, B.L., Hiner, S.L., Neill, P.C., Tierney, W.M. (1986). The effects of positive and negative life changes on the self-reported health status of elderly adults. *Journal of Gerontology*, 41(1), 114-119.

Weissman, M.M., Sholomskas, D., Pottenger, M., Prusoff, B.A., Locke, B.Z. (1977). Assessing depressive symptoms in five psychiatric populations: A validation study. *American Journal of Epidemiology*, Vol 106(3), 203-214.

Yesavage, J.A., Brink, T.L., Rose, T.L,. Lum, O., Huang, V., Adey, M., and Leirer, V.O. (1983). Development and validation of a geriatric depression screening scale: A preliminary report. *Journal of Psychiatric Research*, Vol 17, 31-49.

Chapter Eight

Alcoholism
and the Hispanic Older Adult

Frances K. Lopez-Bushnell, EdD, RNC
Patricia A. Tyra, EdD, RNCS
May Futrell, PhD, RN, FAAN

Editor's Introduction

Lopez-Bushnell, Tyra and Futrell address a social and mental problem within Hispanic cultures (alcoholism) and how it specifically relates to aging.

Previous issues of *Clinical Gerontologist* have included articles and clinical comments on alcoholism in later life:

1982 I (2) 72-73
1985 IV (1) 45-48
1986 V 178, 275, 417, 418, 423, 457, 478, 480
1986 VI (2) 13-15, 135
1987 VII (1) 57-61
1987 VII (2) 3-14, 15-29
1988 VIII (1) 3-26
1989 IX (1) 67-70
1989 IX (2) 65-68
1990 IX (3,4) 67-68, 70, 86, 126

Frances K. Lopez-Bushnell is Assistant Professor, Department of Nursing, University of Lowell, One University Ave., Lowell, MA 01854. Patricia A. Tyra is Associate Professor, Department of Nursing, University of Lowell, and is in private practice, Belmont, MA. May Futrell is Professor, Department of Nursing at the University of Lowell.

as well as reviews of books on this topic.

1983 I (4) 82
1985 III (3) 80-81
1985 IV (1) 59-61
1985 IV (2) 58-59
1987 VII (2) 54-56

Little is known about alcohol use and the prevalence of alcohol abuse among older Hispanics in the United States. The data that are available suggest that this group has a high proportion of heavy drinkers, drunkenness and alcohol related health problems (Caetano, 1986). Culture provides a dominant force in determining health behaviors (Leininger, 1985). The recognition of the Hispanic group's views toward alcohol use and health are necessary prior to planning intervention programs to lower incidence of alcoholism and promote health (Heath, 1978).

Alcoholism is becoming an increasingly apparent problem among the elderly in the United States. According to Futrell et al. (1980), alcohol problems among older people have been underestimated and hidden. The existing data are controversial because of inaccurate methods of detection and the denial of drinking problems by alcoholics and professionals (Tobias et al., 1989; Zimberg, 1985).

The older population seems to be affected by alcohol to a greater degree than the population in general because of compounding physical and mental illness. It is not known whether the elderly drink more or their resistance is decreased. Simon (1980) estimates that 10% of those over age 60 have drinking problems. Zimberg (1974) reported that 10% to 15% of the elderly abuse alcohol in their later years. Schuckit and Miller (1976) state this incidence is even higher for widowers, individuals in poor health and those in difficulty with the police.

As people reach their sixties, the number of medical problems begins to increase, coinciding with the diminished capacity for the body to maintain the level of activity and health experienced at younger ages. A number of health problems follow, many of which appear more frequently with aging, but they also may be symptomatic of alcohol problems (Futrell et al., 1980). The effects from alcohol abuse and alcoholism impairs mental alertness, judgement and physical coordination. In addition reaction time is decreased which increases the risk of falls and accidents. Reported falls of elderly persons have reached epidemic proportions and it is suspected that alcoholism may often be the etiology. Further, heavy drinking can also cause permanent damage to the brain, central nervous system, liver, heart, kidneys, and stomach. The cirrhosis death rate in Mexico is approximately 20 per 100,000 which is almost twice as high as that in the United States (Chavez, 1984). There is a documented high incidence of stomach cancer among the Hispanic population (US Department Health & Human Services, 1985).

Psychological conditions such as depression, memory loss, and mood changes in addition to dramatic changes in economic and social resources, may also indicate a problem with alcohol. However, these are also often associated with aging; as a consequence, alcoholism in the elderly is often missed. Excessive drinking by older persons may be directly related to such external factors as death of a spouse or change in residence. If the elderly can be taught how to cope with these external factors in culturally acceptable ways, the prognosis for successful stress reduction is relatively high (Sandlier, 1980). It would follow that alcohol abuse might be reduced.

What is perceived as frailty, depression, senility, or simply unsteadiness of old age may, in fact be alcoholism. This may mask the diagnostic problems which constitute the greatest barrier to treatment of the elderly alcohol abusing population.

ALCOHOL USE AMONG HISPANIC OLDER PERSONS

Elderly alcoholics fall into three categories. The first group is long-term abusers who have used alcohol excessively throughout life and carry this practice into old age. According to Zimberg (1974) many in this group appear to have personality characteristics similar to younger alcoholics. Today the long-term abuser lives past middle-age because of better nutrition, antibiotics and improved health. The second category includes those elderly who drink late in life to offset stress. Alcohol is used to cope with retirement, lowered income, declining health, and the death of friends and loved ones. Gomberg (1982) suggests that there is also a small but noticeable third category. This group has had a history of episodic heavy drinking, often weekend or binge drinking. The elderly in this group frequently revert to heavy drinking under the stress and loneliness common amongst the elderly in our society.

About 10% to 15% of all elderly seek medical help related to alcohol problems indicating that alcohol consumption among the elderly is a serious issue (National Council on Alcoholism, 1989). Alcohol is a factor in more than 10% of all deaths and 50% of all homicides. The government estimates that approximately 100,000 Americans die from alcohol related causes every year. Amid these statistics, minority groups stand out as frequent victims according to the Secretary's Task Force on Black and Minority Health (US Department of Health & Human Services, 1985). According to Arrendando et al. (1987), Hispanics have higher rates of heavier drinking and problems associated with drinking than the general population. Virtually nothing is known about the Hispanic elderly alcohol abusing person. Although national studies are being conducted to examine the health and nutritional status of Hispanics, as well as studies linking the alcohol use and drinking behaviors of specific groups, surveys in areas with large and more homogeneous Hispanic populations are lacking and badly needed. Geographically limited surveys have the advantage of providing more accurate information about regional differences in drinking habits across Hispanic groups which is important for designing treatment and prevention strategies (Caetano, 1986).

CULTURAL FACTORS AND ALCOHOLISM

Alcoholism in the Hispanic culture has been attributed to numerous factors. For example, one factor which has been noted is Machismo. Machismo is the concept of manly strength and dominance which includes an attitude that a man should be able to drink without showing the effects. This, of course, influences drinking practices. Another cause of drinking may be stress of transition from the native culture to the mainstream United States culture (Alcocer, 1982). A third cause may be the ethnic tradition of male drinking in the Hispanic culture. Poverty is also described in the literature as a contributor to heavy drinking among Hispanics (Yamamato and Steinberg, 1981).

Factors that have been found to influence drinking in other cultures include poverty, prejudice, unemployment (Beltrame and McQueen, 1979) and the stress of integrating into a mainstream culture (Group for the Advancement of Psychiatry, 1989). In contrast, a New Zealand community based sample of elders aged 70 years and older, indicated that with more money alcohol consumption increased (Busby et al., 1988). Drinking may be related to family and friendship. Drunkenness has been found as an acceptable excuse for deviant behavior in some cultures (Ferguson, 2972). Therefore, length of time in the United States may be a factor associated with indicators of alcoholism.

In the Hispanic culture there is evidence that drinking patterns vary with gender. According to Caetano (1986) 13% of Hispanic men report frequent heavy drinking. Only three percent of women report such behavior.

However, information with regard to drinking and gender by cultural groups is sparse.

WORLD VIEW AND PERCEPTION OF HEALTH

One's perception of health may be influenced by his/her world view. Many Hispanic cultures are grounded in the magico-religious paradigm (Boyle and Andrews, 1989). According to the magico-religious paradigm, supernatural forces dominate the world. The actions of God, or the gods, or other supernatural forces of good or evil will determine the fate of the world and those in it. Some cultures believe that the human individual is at the mercy of such forces regardless of his/her behavior while other cultures believe that an individual is punished by gods for his/her wrongdoing. It is expected that people who relate illness to punishment by God, will be less likely to seek medical help than if illness is viewed as a germ that can be destroyed through the use of antibiotics. In the western culture, the Christian Scientists are an example of this paradigm because they believe that physical healing can be effected through prayer alone.

According to the magico-religious paradigm, disease is viewed as the action and result of supernatural forces causing the intrusion of a disease producing foreign body or entrance of a health damaging spirit. The sources of illness in this paradigm are sorcery, breach of taboo, intrusion of a disease object, or a disease-causing spirit, and the loss of soul. One, or any combination, of these sources is given as explanation for the etiology of disease. In the Hispanic culture, *mal ojo* or the "evil eye," the intrusion of a disease causing spirit (Maduro, 1983), is one example of the magico-religious paradigm. Health is seen as a gift or reward from God because it can be seen as a sign of God's special favor for it gives the person the opportunity to resign himself to God's will. Illness is often viewed as God's possession or as a punishment. Alcohol may not be viewed as influencing health in this world view.

The Hispanic people believe in several illnesses based on the magico-religious paradigm including *susto, empacho, caida de la mollera, mal ojo,* and *mal puest.* When an individual experiences a stressful event, the soul or spirit leaves the body and the person experiences restlessness, anorexia, depression, listlessness, disinterest in personal appearance, and the *curandero* or *espiritualista* must perform a ceremony in order to treat the *susto* individual (Hautman and Harrison, 1982). The relationship of the Hispanic elderly's cultural beliefs, drinking patterns, and health status is not known at this time.

CLINICAL ASSESSMENT

Indicators of Alcoholism can be identified by client responses on the 25 question Michigan Alcoholism Screening Test (MAST). The neutral wording on some questions has been reported to detect indicators of alcoholism even with problem drinkers who are reluctant to view themselves in this way and the refusal to respond to questions is very low (Selzer, 1971). The MAST has been shown to have high validity with scores accurately discriminating between alcoholics and nonalcoholics based on independent evidence of problem drinking. A score of three points or less is considered nonalcoholic, a score of four points is suggestive of alcoholism, and a score of five points or more indicates alcoholism. It takes approximately 15 minutes to complete the MAST.

Although Selzer has studied both men and women, his investigations have not been specific to the elderly population or the Hispanic population. Selzer and associates found in their sample of male and female alcoholics ranging in age from 16-72 years (M = 40 years) that the test appeared to be equally effective as a diagnostic tool with men and women (Selzer, Gomberg and Nordhoff, 1979). Willenbring and colleagues from the VA Medical Center in Minneapolis studied the validity of the MAST in 52 hospitalized elderly male alcoholics and 33 nonalcoholic controls (Willenbring, Christensen, Spring, and Rasmussen, 1987). The scores showed high sensitivity (i.e., the ability to correctly identify cases) and specificity (i.e., correct identification of noncases). Dr. Blow from the University of Michigan Alcohol Research Center is in the process of revising the MAST specifically for the elderly.

CONCLUSIONS

Given the known medical and psychological indicators for alcoholism, clinicians have a responsibility to identify these with their clients. Denial by alcoholics of their drinking problem sometimes causes them to refuse assessment, treatment or referrals. That is their individual right. It is the clinician's clinical and ethical responsibility to identify and assess the problem with those clients suspected of alcoholism. The instruments mentioned above may be helpful in such assessments. However, it is hoped that culturally sensitive assessment tools will become available for all clinicians in the near future.

REFERENCES

Agree, E.M. (1988). *A Portrait of Older Minorities*, The AARP Minority Affairs Initiative. Long Beach, California.

Alcocer, A.M. (1982). "Alcohol use and abuse among the Hispanic American population." In: *National Institute on Alcohol Abuse and Alcoholism*. Special Population Issues. Alcohol and Health Monograph No. 4, DHHS Publication No. (ADM) 821193, Washington: Government Printing Office, pp. 361-382.

Arrendando, R., Weddige, R.D., Justice, C.C., & Fitz, J. (1987). "Alcoholism in Mexican-American intervention and treatment." *Hospital Community Psychiatry, 38,* 180-183.

Beltrame, T. and McQueen, D.V. (1979). "Urban and rural Indian drinking patterns: The special case of the Lumbee." *International Journal of Addiction. 14;* 533-548.

Bogue, D.J. (1985). *The Population of the United States Historical Trends and Future Projections.* New York: The Free Press.

Boyle, J.S. and Andrews, M.M. (1989). *Transcultural concepts in nursing care.* Boston: Scott, Foresman/Little, Brown College Division.

Busby, W.J., Campbell, A.J., Borrie, M.J. and Spears, G.F.S. (1988). "Alcohol use in a community-based sample of subjects aged 70 years and older." *The American Geriatrics Society, 36*(4), 301-305.

Caetano, R. (1986). *Patterns and problems of drinking among U.S. Hispanics.* Prepared for the Department of Health and Human Services Task Force on Black and Minority Health. Washington, D.C.

Cairl, R., Pfeiffer, E., Keller, D., Burke, H., & Samis, H. (1983). "An evaluation of the reliability and validity of the functional assessment inventory." *Journal of the American Geriatrics Society, 31,* 607-612.

Chavez, R.L. (1984). "Doctors, *curanderos,* and *brujas*: Health care delivery and Mexican immigrants in San Diego." *Medical Anthropology Quarterly, 15*(2), 31-37.

"Elderly Hispanics face greater poverty." (1989, September 14). *The Boston Globe,* p. 22.

Ferguson, F.N. (1972). "A Stake in Society: Its Relevance to Response by Navajo Alcoholics in a Treatment Program." Ph.D. dissertation. University of North Carolina, Chapel Hill.

Futrell, M., Brovender, S., McKinnon-Mullet, E., and Brower, H., (1980). *Primary health care of the older adult.* North Situate, MA: Duxbury Press.

Gomberg, S. (1982). "Alcohol and the elderly: An overview." *Aging program letter, 1* (4), Omni Reports, p. 2.

Group for the Advancement of Psychiatry (1989). "Suicide and ethnicity in the United States." New York: Brunner/Mazel.

Hautman, M.A. and Harrison, J.K. (1982). "Health beliefs and practices in a middle income Anglo-American neighborhood." *Advances in Nursing Science, 4* (3), 49-64.

Heath, D.B. (1978). "The sociocultural model of alcohol use: Problems and prospects." *Journal of Operational Psychiatry, 9* (1), 55-66.

Kincannon, C.L. (1980). *Census of the Population.* U.S. Department of Commerce: Bureau of the Census Vol. 1.

Leininger, M.M. (1985). "Transcultural care diversity and universality: A theory of nursing." *Nursing and Health Care, 6* (4), 209-212.

Maduro, R. (1983). "Curanderismo and Latino views of disease and curing." *The Journal of Medicine, 139* (6), 869-874.

National Council on Alcoholism Inc. (1989). *Factors on alcoholism and alcohol related problems.* New York: National Council on Alcoholism.

Pfeiffer, E. (1975). "A short portable mental status questionnaire for the assessment of organic brain deficit in elderly patients." *Journal of the American Geriatrics Society, 23,* 433-441.

Sandlier, M. (1980). *The invisible alcoholics: Women and alcohol use in America.* New York: McGraw-Hill Book Co.

Schuckit, M., and Miller P. (1976). "Men and women's responses to the Michigan alcoholism screening test." *Journal of Studies on Alcohol, 40,* 502-504.

Selzer, M., Gomberg, E., and Nordhoff, J. (1979). "Men and women's responses to the Michigan alcoholism screening test." *Journal of Studies on Alcohol, 40,* 502-504.

Simon, A. (1980). "The neuroses, personality disorders, alcoholism, drug use and misuses, and crime in the aged." In Birren, J.E., Sloane, R.B. (Eds.) *Handbook of Mental Health and Aging* (pp. 653-670). Englewood Cliffs: Prentice-Hall Publishers.

Tobias, C., Lippmann, S., Perry, R., Oropilla, and Embry, C.K. (1989). "Alcoholism in the elderly: How to spot and treat a problem the patient wants to hide." *Post-Graduate Medicine, 86* (4), 67-79.

U.S. Department of Health and Human Services. (1985). *Report of the Secretary's Task Force on Black and Minority Health* (Volume VII: Chemical Dependency and Diabetes) Washington, DC: U.S. Government Printing Office.

Usui, W. (1989). "Challenges in the development of ethnogerontology." *The Gerontologist, 29,* 566-568.

Willenbring, M., Christensen, K., Spring, W., and Rasmussen, R. (1987). "Alcoholism screening in the elderly." *Journal of the American Geriatrics Society, 35,* 864-869.

Yamamato, J. and Steinberg, A. (1981). "Ethic, racial, and social class factors in mental health." *Journal of the National Medical Association, 73,* 231-240.

Zimberg, S. (1974). "The elderly alcoholic." *Gerontologist, 14* (4), 221-224.

Zimberg, S. (1985). "Treating the older alcoholic." *Geriatric Medicine Today, 4* (1), 68-77.

Chapter Nine

Assessing Impairment Among Hispanic Elderly: Biomedical and Ethnomedical Perspectives

Judith Freidenberg, PhD
Ivonne Z. Jiménez-Velazquez, MD

Editor's Introduction

Freidenberg and Jiménez-Velazquez demonstrate how to do a comprehensive assessment of patients: functional, cognitive, emotional and medical, from a sensitive, ethno-cultural perspective. The result is not only an interesting statistical table, but also case studies illustrating interactions between "biomedical" and "ethnomedical" conditions.

Judith Freidenberg is Assistant Professor, Community Medicine and Geriatrics, Mount Sinai School of Medicine, City University of New York. Ivonne Z. Jiménez-Velazquez is Assistant Professor, Internal Medicine and Geriatrics, University of Puerto Rico School of Medicine and Adjunct Assistant Professor of Geriatrics, Mount Sinai School of Medicine, City University of New York.

This research was supported in part by a grant from the National Institute on Aging (1-R21-AGO-702701) to the senior author, whose support the authors gratefully acknowledge. The authors are indebted as well to Robert Butler, MD for providing the departmental structure and the personal support for our collaboration; to Michael Mulvihill, MPH for collaborating effectively in all phases of the larger study; to Judith Bornstein for her assistance in coding the interviews; and to Myrna Lewis, MSW, T. L. Brink, PhD for helpful editorial suggestions to earlier versions of this paper. Mr. Ramón López and Ms. Olga Achinelly are also due thanks for their assistance in the preparation of the manuscript.

INTRODUCTION

Assessing impairment among Hispanic elderly is an important task, for both researchers and practitioners (Markides & Mindel, 1987; Torres-Gil, 1986; Commonwealth Fund Commission, 1989; Butler & Lewis, 1991). In this chapter, we report on an approach which, by combining a biomedical and an ethnomedical perspective, attempts to render assessment of impairment in the community more culturally sensitive (Hahn & Kleinman, 1983).

DESCRIPTION OF THE STUDY

Our approach was developed by an interdisciplinary team consisting of a geriatrician and an anthropologist as part of a larger ethnographic study of the health seeking process.

The ethnographic study of the health seeking process was based on 48 elderly Hispanic informants currently residing in East Harlem, New York. In order to be sensitive to the demographic variability of this population, Dr. Freidenberg identified a sample equally distributed by age, sex, living arrangements and use of mainstream care. Since the latter variable was thought to be crucial for the understanding of utilization and access issues, informants were recruited using a variety of sources: hospital clinics, senior citizen centers, nutrition programs, advocacy programs, private physicians' offices, housing projects for the elderly, herbal stores (*botánicas*), churches, and institutions and agencies which serve the East Harlem elderly. Presentations were given at each of these locales to explain the research goals and enlist the agencies' cooperation in referring people appropriate to the study. A large number of people were approached until the sample size was obtained.

During the course of staff meetings related to this project with an epidemiologist and a geriatrician, we became deeply aware that clinicians worked with *patients* who came to the institution, as part of their socialization to the professional medical system, whereas the anthropologist attempted to understand the *person* within his/her social and cultural milieu, regardless of whether the person was or would become a patient. This provided the rationale for having the geriatrician and the anthropologist visit the households together to study impairment from a clinical and an ethnographic perspective. Additionally, the anthropologist's long-term involvement of the with the sample provided the study with both longitudinal and cross-sectional data.

An interview schedule was developed for use with the 40 individuals who agreed to participate in the study. The schedule combined existing assessment impairment instruments, translated and validated for Spanish-speaking populations, with questions related to help-seeking behavior. Dr. Jiménez-Velazquez conducted most of the interviews while Dr. Freidenberg recorded the anthropological aspects of the setting, both those observed at the interview as well as those known through long-term ethnographic fieldwork. After the interview, we summarized the case from a clinical and a population perspective. The interview time was approximately two hours and was conducted in Spanish.

The work on which we report here, therefore, combines information on impairment gathered from a biomedical and an ethnomedical perspective.

Biomedical Perspective

1. *Functional assessment*: Fourteen questions on Activities of Daily Living-ADL-and Instrumental Activities of Daily Living-IADL-(Duke University, 1978), are currently in use as part of the intake clinical interview at the Coffey Elderly Clinic at Mount Sinai Medical Center, administered by the Department of Geriatrics. These instruments are used in this study to ensure comparability between a patient and a community population. The version translated into Spanish by the Family Guidance Center in Florida, validated with a population of Cuban elders, was selected over other alternatives. A section on use and need of aids, developed at Mount Sinai Geriatric Clinic, was also included.

The functional assessment section was modified by Dr. Freidenberg to cover the experience of the problems, the nature of the help received and the timing between perceiving needs and meeting them. Specifically, questions dealt with the informant's description of the problem and its causes, frequency in receiving help, residence of the helper and reciprocity in helping relationships. These questions were translated by Dr. Freidenberg with feedback from Dr. Jiménez-Velazquez.

2. *Cognitive assessment*: The Mini-Mental State Examination (MMSE), incorporated in the National Institute of Mental Health Diagnostic Interview Schedule, was selected (Folstein et al., 1975), for its epidemiological significance in cross-cultural research, particularly with Hispanics (Escobar et al., 1986). The instrument was translated into Spanish by Dr. Jiménez-Velazquez, checked for ethnomethodological soundness with Dr. Jagendra Jutagir and the tongue twister revised on semantic appropriateness. Dr. Jiménez-Velazquez is at present using this instrument for the purposes of validation with a sample of Puerto Rican elderly currently living in San Juan, Puerto Rico.

3. *Emotional assessment*: We selected a Spanish version of the Geriat-

ric Depression Scale (GDS), designed specifically for rating depression in the elderly (Yesavage and Brink, 1983). This version, at the time of the study, was under validation at the University of Puerto Rico by Dr. Juan A. Rosado-Matos (personal communication), in order to compare populations of Puerto Ricans on the mainland and on the island at a later date.

4. *Medical Assessment*: Among the medical aspects of the study Dr. Jiménez-Velazquez recorded information about the patients' hearing and visual acuities, their ability to walk, and their blood pressures.

Ethnomedical Perspective

During the course of the interview study, generated by ethnographic fieldwork, informants were asked about patterns of health-seeking, utilization of professional, popular and folk sectors of care and about experienced difficulties in accessing formal sources of care. Information gathered on the social, economic and environmental circumstances affecting their daily lives throughout the ethnographic study provided an explanatory framework for the cross-sectional data and also validated ethnographic data. Three issues addressed here are: (1) worrisome health problems experienced during the year preceding the interview, (2) regularity of utilization of medical care and (3) knowledge and use of social services, home attendant agencies and nutrition programs. Data on those issues is derived from informants' reports on their health status and the actions they took when they thought there was something they could do in response to their worrisome health concerns.

RESULTS

We analyzed the data in two steps. First, we classified informants by degree of impairment from both perspectives and then compared the congruence between the two data sets. The functional assessment questionnaire was administered to 39 of 40 persons. It shows that 27/39 (69%) of the informants were in the normal to mild functional range, as expected in a community of non-institutionalized elderly. Twelve of thirty-nine (31%) were living at home with moderate to severe functional impairments.

The Geriatric Depression Scale was answered completely by 32 of 40 persons at the time of the study. It suggests that 11/32 (34%) are in what we determined to be high risk for depression, which may be affecting their performance in the other assessment tools and also in their personal conceptualization of health status and needs. Twenty-one of thirty-two (66%) showed a lower risk for depressions which may indicate their high capacity for adjustment to their level of poverty, illness (or impairment) and social disadvantage related to their minority status.

The scale for cognitive assessment (Folstein, Mini-Mental) has been extensively used and discussed in the literature, but required some adjustment to be adequately understood by a mainly Puerto Rican population. It was administered after a thorough discussion with Dr. Raj Jutagir (Neuropsychologist at Mount Sinai School of Medicine Geriatrics Clinic). It shows that 13/40 (32.5%) have a considerable cognitive impairment, which suggests a sub-group that may actually require more help and social support in order to continue living and "functioning" at home. This may also be altering their perception of health status and needs. Twenty-one of forty (67.5%) showed mild to no impairment.

A scale was designed specifically for this study to help the clinician determine the level of physical ability to function independently at home, including a marker of disease (HBP). We found that 23/38 (60%) of our sample were classified as moderate to severely impaired (as determined by 2 or more positive indicators), which is not surprising in an elderly minority population like ours. This high level of impairment may be contributing to difficulties coping and maintaining an adequate functional status at home.

The second step in our analysis involved grouping our sample by biomedical and ethnomedical perspectives. Using each of the health status measures, we studied the degrees of impairment and explored the extent to which the biomedical and ethnomedical perspectives converged or diverged.

Table I clearly shows that the biomedical perspective on the person's health status does not always coincide with the person's perceptions.

In a second step, we analyzed the extent to which health needs were unaddressed by either the medical or non-medical systems. We presumed scoring severe in either or both the biomedical or ethnomedical perspectives was a clear indication of being in need of assistance. That assistance, in terms of our clinical and social assessment, but also based on the ethnographic understanding of this population, was conceptualized as medical (doctors, nurses, and other medical-related personnel) and non-medical (home care/attendant, social and nutrition services).

An analysis of impairment by use of medical and non-medical facilities showed that health status is unrelated to utilization patterns. This points to factors that might be affecting access, which exceeds the scope of this paper.

In order to provide more clarity to the argument, we will exemplify with a case for each category. These cases encompass the clinician's ren-

CONGRUENCE OF BIOMEDICAL AND ETHNOMEDICAL MODELS OF IMPAIRMENT

I—FUNCTIONAL ASSESSMENT   II—COGNITIVE ASSESSMENT

BIOMEDICAL MODEL

I—FUNCTIONAL ASSESSMENT

ETHNOMEDICAL MODEL	MILD TO MODERATE	MODERATE TO SEVERE
MILD TO MODERATE	1 15 28 45 3 16 31 48 4 19 37 8 21 38 12 23 40 14 27 44	11 43
MODERATE TO SEVERE	5 36 9 10 18 22 30	2 29 6 35 7 39 17 42 20 25

II—COGNITIVE ASSESSMENT

ETHNOMEDICAL MODEL	MILD TO MODERATE	MODERATE TO SEVERE
MILD TO MODERATE	1 14 26 3 15 27 4 16 28 8 19 31 11 21 38 12 23	37 40 43 44 45 48
MODERATE TO SEVERE	2 25 5 30 10 36 17 42 20 22	6 39 7 9 18 29 35

III-EMOTIONAL ASSESSMENT   IV-PHYSICAL ASSESSMENT

BIOMEDICAL MODEL

III-EMOTIONAL ASSESSMENT

ETHNOMEDICAL MODEL	MILD TO MODERATE	MODERATE TO SEVERE
MILD TO MODERATE	1 16 44 4 23 45 8 26 11 27 14 28 15 43	12 19 21 31 40 48
MODERATE TO SEVERE	2 36 7 22 25 29 35	10 17 20 30 39 42

IV-PHYSICAL ASSESSMENT

ETHNOMEDICAL MODEL	MILD TO MODERATE	MODERATE TO SEVERE
MILD TO MODERATE	3 19 4 23 8 26 12 31 14 45 15	1 37 11 38 16 40 21 43 27 44 38 48
MODERATE TO SEVERE	10 18 25 30	2 22 5 29 6 35 7 36 9 39 17 42

The numbers in each cell represent the informant's numbers, as given in the original anthropological study.

The authors acknowledge Lloyd A. LeZotte, Jr., MD, PhD, who helped in the preparation of this table.

dering of health status, interpreted against the background of the general population, as well as the anthropologist's reading of perceived health appraisal in a social and environmental context. Viewing the cases in this light provides a better grasp of health status with clear implications for interventions geared to addressing areas of need.

CASES

Case 1: Mild Biomedical with Mild Ethnomedical (#4)

This is a 68 year old male patient, single and living alone, known as a "hard worker." He is very active, has a good character and a sense of humor and is actually the "super" at a building. He was able to do all ADL's, housechores, and other items included in the functional assessment instrument without help. He denied having any specific needs. He denied medical illness and was considered a reliable informant. During the medical assessment, no impairments were found. He was well oriented, although his immediate memory was impaired. The emotional assessment showed no evidence of depression related to his present status, but a concern for the future was clearly stated.

In this case, the client's perceptions of health status were adequately confirmed by the clinician as well as shared by the anthropologist. Case 1 had only one health concern: asthma, which he thinks is brought about by an allergy. When it got worse two years ago, he decided to consult with a physician right away. He made this decision by himself and went alone. He knows about social services, nutrition and home care services but does not use them.

Case 2: Severe Biomedical with Severe Ethnomedical (#39)

An 80 year old female patient who lives by herself, but is cared for by a 24 hour home attendant. She is unable to walk without help, and has worsened in the last year. She is able to eat, use the phone and take her medications on her own, but requires help for all other functional items questioned. She confides that, as she has become more needy, her character has changed. Her medical problems consist of bone pains [arthritis], inability to walk, angina, fatigue, and difficulty moving her arms. Patients' needs are referred to as multiple. Some needs are addressed — for example, she has a shower chair — while others are unaddressed — for example, has been waiting for a new dental prosthesis for the last two years. The patient complains that she is not capable even of writing a letter to a friend. Her self-esteem is very low as she says: "I have no value. I am not worth two cents." The patient expresses she likes to read, but her vision is actually impaired and not corrected with eyeglasses. Her audition has decreased. Mini-mental test showed considerable impairment, because her immediate and recent memory were inadequate, but she was well-oriented and her mind seemed clear to the clinician. Emotional assessment showed high risk for depression which could be related to her physical and functional impairment.

Case 2 was worried about the following health conditions last year: heart, asthma, arthritis, "presion emotiva" (circulation) problems, vision problems and "intestinal obstruction" (constipation). Of those, she was most worried about the vision problems, arthritis and intestinal obstruction (constipation) although it is her heart condition and asthma that bother her chronically. Her symptoms are pain in her leg and arm muscles, inability to walk, swollen feet, almost total loss of vision, and eye itching. Lately, she reported her intestinal obstruction (constipation) got worse and she thought she should do something about it. She believes the intestinal obstruction (constipation) results from her inability to move while her vision problems result from an eye operation which has done more harm than good. She consulted with a physician, who hospitalized her and performed an enema. She also consulted a botanist (at a "botánica") who supplied herbs. At the time of the study, she was most concerned about asthma, headaches and blood pressure. She was affected greatly by her sister's death, which she believes to be the cause of her high blood pressure. When she had dizzy spells her home attendant called her daughter who called the police. They, in turn, called the ambulance and she was taken to the emergency room. She was then referred back to her regular physician. She also discussed her concerns with her full-time home attendant. She consults the medical system with regularity. She uses alternative systems of care simultaneously. In the past, she was able to read cards, light candles to the saints, go to the botánica, and make promises at church. Now that she is partly disabled, she uses only home remedies such as ruda, alcanfor and alcohol to alleviate arthritis. She also prays every night and carries an image of "Angel de la Guardia de Mercedes," which she takes off only to take baths and which she buys also at the botánica. She has a full-time home attendant, knows about social services yet does not use them and has knowledge of nutrition programs. Case 2 was born in Cuba and shares her apartment with the home attendant (who spends weekends at home in the Bronx) and a niece who is not there all the time. She believes that by being quiet and compliant she also helps her helper. Being almost unable to walk and seeing her living room "converted into a clinic'' makes her feel quite depressed; being unable to cook makes her perceive herself as worthless and uncomfortably dependent.

Case 3: Severe Biomedical and Mild Ethnomedical (#43)

This is an 87 year old male who lives with his wife. He is able to walk at home with a cane but cannot go out because his legs are "too heavy." He is continent, able to feed himself, prepare some food and make telephone calls.He states he could take his medications by himself but his wife does not let him. She also pampers him in several other ways. His illness and physical impairments make it impossible for him to live independently. His vision and audition are impaired and he is unable to get a hearing aid due to financial difficulties. The mini-mental test showed some degree of dementia or moderate cognitive impairment.

This elderly male is very sick; his functional capacity is markedly diminished and he has been followed at the "Joints Disease Hospital" for severe arthritis. However, his faith in God is very strong and his emotional ability to cope is remarkable. The emotional status instrument showed a low risk for depression.

Yet this patient considers himself as only mildly impaired. Case 3 is mostly concerned about "life worries." This is a "hot" condition that makes him feel desperate. Although this condition is chronic, he does not think it is serious and so "lets it pass" since he believes this problem is due to aging and cannot be helped. He only consults with his wife who thinks he should just remain calm, which he will continue to do "till God allows it." Following her advice has made him feel better but he also takes other actions to alleviate discomfort. He buys home remedies at a "Botánica"; particularly relevant to his condition is tea of MEJORANA, to help him sleep and for stomach upsets. When he gets very tense, his wife massages him with BEN-GAY, a cream he obtains at the pharmacy. Unfailingly, they both light candles to the Power of God, once a month. They pray to God with much faith. As he wakes up, he reads the Bible. He consults a physician only for particular problems because "they ask you a lot of questions and they do nothing. You waste your time. I want the Doctor to tell me what I have, not to ask me. They just told me last time that I should stay calm — "que lo cogiera suave" — and return for another appointment. They only give you another appointment because they get paid for it." This man does not know about home attendant, social or nutritional services.

Case 4: Mild Biomedical and Severe Ethnomedical (#30)

This 61 year old male avoided visual contact during the course of the interview and preferred to sit with his back to the clinician. He lives with his wife and they have a home attendant for four hours per day, 5 days per week. Patient claims independence in all ADL's but admitted he required help to clean the house. His wife helps to pay the bills. Patient complains of severe financial problems.

Although this client carries several medical diagnoses — such as arterial hypertension, heart disease, diabetes mellitus and peptic ulcer disease — he was medically stable at the time of the study and not physically impaired. However, as could be clearly observed and confirmed by means of the Yesavage questionnaire, the patient admitted to having a severe depression. He confided that his physician did not treat him because "he couldn't prescribe more medications for me." His cognitive status was not impaired but his health status and needs were interpreted as markedly impaired and high, respectively, under the influence of a severe depressive state.

Case 4's health concerns last year were ulcer, diabetes, heart, arthritis and "despair." The one that he feels the most discomfort with is diabetes. He explains it is a "hot" condition because "you feel depressed, you don't feel calm, no matter what happens, you feel bad." This happens to him most of the time. Last year, when his diabetes got high, he decided to go to the doctor, but in reality he was seeking comfort for his low feelings. He said: "The despair sticks to you to such an extent that you look at the clinic to alleviate the feeling, you go to a doctor to get medicine." He only asks his wife for advice but he also prays because going to the doctor has not alleviated his symptoms. He also talks to a priest, whom he feels very close to, "like a brother. You go to the priest for spiritual problems, and to the doctor for material problems. When you are depressed, you need to seek God first and then everything follows. But also diabetes depress you. The priest told me to pray to God to recuperate my calmness." He follows instructions from the physician and the priest, as well as taking teas — such as orange and cinnamon — that help him fall asleep. Although the doctor, whom he consults regularly, gives him an appointment every three months, he would like to go when he feels the need for it. He uses a home attendant four hours a day. He also uses social services and nutrition programs, the latter two at a Senior Citizen Center that he attends almost daily.

DISCUSSION

Comprehensive assessment of elderly patients in clinical settings is becoming essential for optimal clinical management (Applegate, 1990). In the community, evaluations need to be performed by a team with a clinical and a social science background to screen for cases that need medical and/or social interventions before they deteriorate to the point when institutionalization is unavoidable.

Medical labelling and the patient's perception of impairment can diverge. While the biomedical view labels impairment, the ethnomedical perspective provides the social and cultural context of *coping* with impairment. The biomedical health status indicators do not predict utilization of either the medical or the non-medical health care system. The practitioner, who combines a preventive with a curative outlook, should develop field approaches and refine methodologies to assess impairment among the non-institutionalized elderly and provide case-management interventions to care for the elderly in their homes. The policy maker must build on this and design community outreach programs and health education ventures designed for practitioner and client alike. For the Hispanic elderly, who are extremely vulnerable and under-utilize medical and non-medical facilities, the design of interventions that emerges from knowledge gained on community samples could be one of the difficult, yet unavoidable, challenges of the 1990's.

REFERENCES

HISPANIC ELDERLY

Commonwealth Fund Commission (1989). Poverty and Poor Health among Elderly Hispanic Americans: Baltimore, MD.

Community Service Society (1987). Poverty in New York City 1980-1985. New York: Community Service Society.

Gann, L.H. & Duignan, P.S. (1986). The Hispanics in the United States Boulder, Colorado: Westview Press.

Markides, K. & Mindel, M. (1987). Aging and Ethnicity. Newbury Park, CA: Sage.

Sotomayor, M. & Curiel, H. (Eds.) (1988). Hispanic Elderly: A Cultural Signature Edinburg, TX: Pan American University Press.

Torres-Gil, F. (1986). Hispanics in an Aging Society. New York: Carnegie Corporation.

ASSESSMENT OF ELDERLY NEEDS

Applegate, W.E. (1990). Instruments for the Functional Assessment of Older Patients, New Eng Jour of Med, Vol. 322, No. 17.

Butler, R.N. and Lewis, M.I. (1991). Aging and Mental Health St. Louis, Mo: Mosby.

Commonwealth Fund Commission (1987). Old, Alone and Poor: A Plan for Reducing Poverty among Elderly People. Baltimore, MD.

ASSESSMENT OF IMPAIRMENT

I. COGNITIVE

Escobar, J. et al. (1986). Use of the Mini-Mental State Examination in a Community Population of Mixed Ethnicity; Cultural and Linguistic Artifacts. *Journal of Nervous and Mental Disease, 174*(10).

Folstein, M.F. et al. (1975). Mini-Mental State: A Practical Method for Grading the Cognitive State of Patients for the Clinician. *Journal of Psychiatric Research. 12*:189-198.

II. MOOD AND DEPRESSION

Yesavage J. & Brink T.L. (1983) Development and Validation of a Geriatric Depression Screening Scale: A Preliminary Report Journal of Psychiatric Research, *17*:37-49.

III. PHYSICAL

Lichtenstein, M.H. et al.(1988). Validation of Screening Tools for Identifying Hearing-Impaired Elderly in Primary Care. *JAMA, 259*:2875-2878.

Mathias, S. et al. (1986). Balance in Elderly Patient. Archives Phys. Med. Rehabil., *67*:387-389.

Ventry I.M. & Weinstein B. (1983). Identification of Elderly People with Hearing Problems. *ASHA*: 37-42.

IV. FUNCTIONAL

Duke University Center for the Study of Aging and Human Development (1978). Multidimensional Functional Assessment: The OARS Methodology, a Manual Durham, N.C.

BIOMEDICAL/ETHNOMEDICAL MODELS

Frankenberg, R. (1988). Essays for the Development of Critical Medical Anthropology. *Medical Anthropology Quarterly, 2*(4):324-337.

Hahn, R. & Kleinman, A. (1983). Biomedical Practice and Anthropological Theory: Frameworks and Directions. *Ann. Rev. Anthrop. 12*:305-33.

Menendez, E. L. (1981). Poder, Estratificacion y Salud: Analisis de las Condiciones Sociales y Economicas de la Enfermedad en Yucatan Mexico: Siglo XXI.

Young, A. (1982). The Anthropologies of Illness and Sickness Ann. Rev. *Anthropol. 11*:257-85.

HEALTH SEEKING PROCESS

Chrisman, N. & Kleinman, A. (1980). Health Beliefs and Practices among American Ethnic Groups. In S. Thorenstorm (Ed.). Harvard Encyclopedia of American Ethnic Groups Cambridge, MA: Harvard University Press.

Garrison V. (1977). Doctor, Espiritista or Psychiatrist? Health Seeking Behavior in a Puerto Rican Neighborhood of New York City. *Medical Anthropology, 1*(2):65-179

Kleinman, A. et al. (1978). Culture, Illness and Care: Clinical Lessons from Anthropologic and Cross-Cultural Research. *Annals of Internal Medicine 88*:251-258.

Zola, I.K. (1973). Pathways to the Doctor—From Person to Patient. *Social Science and Medicine, vol. 7*:677-689.

Chapter Ten

Treating the Sequelae of a Curse in Elderly Mexican-Americans

George Gafner, MSW, ACSW
Stephane Duckett, PhD

Editor's Introduction

Gafner reiterates the need for sensitivity to ethno-cultural themes, especially the Hispanic elder's belief in folk healing (*curanderismo*) and the power of curses (*brujerismo*).

Faith healing, folk medicine and superstitions have not been the focus of previous articles in *Clinical Gerontologist*, but religion has been a topic:

1987 VII (1) 86-87
1988 VIII (1) 89-91
1990 X (2) 93-98
1990 X (2) 116

and so has pastoral care:

1983 II (1) 80
1984 II (4) 37-49
1985 III (4) 98-99
1985 IV (1) 97-98
1988 VII (3/4) 94-96

George Gafner is coordinator of the family therapy training program at the V.A. Medical Center, Tucson, AZ. Stephane Duckett is a psychologist at the Bryn Mawr Rehabilitation Hospital, Malvern, PA.

A version of this paper was presented at the American Society on Aging Annual Meeting, New Orleans, LA, March 18, 1991.

WITCHCRAFT, FAITH AND HEALING:
TREATING THE SEQUELAE OF A CURSE
IN ELDERLY MEXICAN-AMERICANS

The Case of Mr. and Mrs. Esquivel

Mr. and Mrs. Esquivel (not their real name), a Mexican-American couple in their late sixties, were seen one time together in family therapy. The couple denied a relationship problem and noted that the presenting problem was difficulty dealing with harassment of a *bruja*, or witch, who lived in the neighborhood. Harassment, which had gone on for many years, included throwing stones on their roof at night, breaking windows, and leaving items in their driveway such as dead toads and wooden crosses smeared with human waste.

Prior to the second appointment the couple were eating steaks that they had barbequed in their backyard when Mr. Esquivel aspirated a piece of meat. He was taken to the V.A. Medical Center where he was placed on a ventilator. After two weeks of medical complications his condition worsened and he was near death, but still conscious. His wife, who claimed skills as a *curandera*, performed a healing ritual on her husband in the intensive care unit. The next morning he died, ostensibly from the sequelae of the *bruja*'s curse.

One would expect subsequent therapy with the widow to involve complicated grief and increased susceptibility to the malevolent influences of the *bruja*; however, her husband's death appeared to free Mrs. Esquivel to assertively confront the *bruja* for the first time.

The Case of Mr. Molina

Mr. Molina (not his real name) was referred to the family therapist because it was believed the therapists's ability to speak Spanish might access the presumed cultural component of the patient's depression. Mr. Molina, age 76, was a resident of the V.A.'s nursing home. Staff complained that the patient was refusing to eat and made remarks about wishing he were dead. Furthermore, he would frequently mention witchcraft, and said that he saw Satan standing by his bed at night. The patient had a 20-year history of Parkinson's disease, which was now severe. He could not walk or transfer on his own and he required assistance in most activities of daily living. However, he was cognitively intact.

Mr. Molina claimed he was first cursed at age 12 when he was fishing in a river in rural Arizona. A local *brujo*, or male witch, working through two Caucasian boys who accompanied Molina to the river, put a tranquilizing agent into his soda pop and afterward beat him with a baseball bat. He did not seek treatment after the incident, and eventually considered the matter closed.

More than 50 years passed before he was cursed a second time. In the interim Mr. Molina was an amateur boxer before serving as an infantryman in Europe during WW II, and he later retired from a job as a laborer in the copper mines. During his younger years he drank heavily, and by the time of the second curse his ex-wife and six children had little contact with him.

He lived alone in low-income housing and Parkinson's had started to limit his activities. One day while walking outside the effects of a curse caused a serious fall and he recalled that his body was "as rigid as stone." Treatment from a *curandera* provided immediate relief; however, the effects of this curse were still evident 12 years later when he was referred for depression.

Folk Medicine in the Southwest

Folk medicine encompasses beliefs and practices that permeate every society to some degree (Marsh, Hentges, 1988). *Curanderismo*, the Mexican-American form of folk healing, has been practiced in Mexico and the southwestern United States since the Spanish Conquest, when medieval medicine and Catholicism were blended with indigenous Indian medicine.

Major components of *curanderismo* include (1) the belief that God heals through *curanderos*, or people with the *don*, or special gift; (2) the existence of a group of naturalistic folk conditions amenable to cure such as *empacho*, or blocked intestine; (3) a belief in the existence of mystical disease, such as *susto* (fright, or lost soul), and *dano* or *mal puesto* (hex or curse); (4) a belief in three levels of health and illness—the material, spiritual and mental; and (5) the use of medicinal herbs and specific rituals in healing. (Kiev, 1964; Marsh and Hentges, 1988; and Romeo, 1990.)

Estimates of utilization of *curanderismo* vary. Meredith (1984) found adherence to depend on locally prevailing economic and social conditions; however, Torres (1983) found that utilization in many communities might be much higher. Utilization might involve either exclusive or partial treatment by a *curandero*. With partial treatment, a patient with arthritis, for example, might visit her physician, fill her prescriptions, and then visit the neighborhood *curandero*, who could instruct her to be sure to take the big red pill, but only with spearmint tea. If the same elderly patient visited a different *curandero* (curandero is a male healer, while curandera denotes female) her treatment might include the passing of a raw egg over painful joints while he recites the Apostles' Creed. Another *curandero*, who specializes in being a *sobador*, or masseur, might massage the patient with an aromatic oil and instruct her to apply bee ointment at home. The *curandero* might also decline to treat, recommending treatment by a physician instead.

Curanderos are utilized for numerous reasons. Patients do not have to travel great distances and they do not have to call ahead for an appointment. Furthermore, there are no complicated forms to complete and it is all right if patients cannot pay. If they can pay, either with money or in trade, that is all right, too. The *curandero* believes in his diagnosis and treatment and does not have to order laboratory tests and x-rays. Instead, he turns to meaningful sources of strength such as the saints and God. Where a physician's office or emergency room is usually cold and technological, the *curandero* embraces, shelters and warms.

The appeal of the *curandero* also lies in the common language and culture in which patients and their families have a shared set of assumptions about cause of illness and its treatment; in the recognition of the profound effect of emotions on health; in the expectant hope of the patient, as the *curandero* enters his personal world with structured emotional closeness; in the high prestige of the healer; and in the warm personal relationship between *curandero* and patient. (Prince, 1981; Torres, 1983)

Curanderos commonly treat *susto*, meaning loss of spirit or shock or fright. This condition, along with its more serious form, *espanto*, can manifest itself as traumatic neurosis, or depression and anxiety. *Susto* can be caused by an upsetting event such as a nightmare or a fall from bed. *Susto*, like *dano* and *ojo* (hex), can be brought about by someone who engages the services of a *brujo*, or witch.

DISCUSSION

Mr. and Mrs. Esquivel

In the cases of both Mr. Molina and the Esquivels, it is important to examine the function of the behavior and the cultural context. Mr. and Mrs. Esquivel, married in 1965, the second marriage for both. Shortly after they married, Mr. Esquivel was shot during an attempted robbery of his restaurant and he was left paralyzed from the waist down. Mrs. Esquivel subsequently sold her retail business and spent the next twenty-five years as a devoted caregiver in an unhappy marriage. As Mr. Esquivel was impotent, his wife carried on an affair throughout the marriage.

The curse is best understood within the context of the unhappy marriage and Mrs. Esquivel's world view. Both Esquivels verified the stones banging on their roof and other harassment, although it was more of a problem for Mrs. Esquivel, who dwelled on it to the exclusion of any other topic. The couple were convinced that Mr. Esquivel's family hired the *bruja* to carry out the harassment, as Mr. Esquivel's mother and other family members were displeased with his choice of wife and blamed her for the paraplegic's problems.

Mrs. Esquivel had always maintained a world view that was laced with superstition. She arbitrarily divided the world into good and evil. Her cultural delusion was limited to her own situation, as she was otherwise appropriate and functioned competently. As she and her husband remained focussed on the *bruja's* harassment, they were distracted from their own emotional distancing and conflict avoidance. An additional function of the delusion for Mrs. Esquivel was the assuagement of her guilt over the affair and regret for years wasted as a caregiver in an unhappy marriage. If Mr. Esquivel had not died and had the couple remained in therapy, the relationship problem would have inevitably displaced the curse as the chief complaint.

Because her delusion served a definite purpose, she was well defended and had plausible reasons for remaining in her situation whenever the therapist or her daughter (who lived in California) suggested she move or otherwise extricate herself from her stressful situation.

In the intensive care unit, Mrs. Esquivel employed holy water, a rosary and prayer as she passed a yellow chile over her husband shortly before his death. In the end, she could say she had always tried her very best. After her husband's death, she showed no signs of grief. Her mood brightened, her anxiety disappeared, and she had a higher fence built around her yard. Suddenly the harassment lessened dramatically. She no longer perseverated on the evil doing of the bruja, and she spoke fondly of moving to California to be nearer her lover and daughter. Also, she declined further therapy appointments, as she said she felt much better.

Mr. Molina

While mental health treatment for Mrs. Esquivel was passive and supportive, Mr. Molina's treatment involved active intervention. Because of the Parkinson patient's weakness and fatigue, the therapist chose to alternate brief sessions with reading Mr. Molina stories in Spanish about Mexican folklore, and especially stories about *curanderos* and *brujas*. Reading and discussion about witchcraft and healing fall into the realm of paradoxical therapy and stand in marked contrast to the staff in the nursing home who discouraged talk about witchcraft.

Early in therapy Mr. Molina spoke about the second curse that happened to him in his early sixties when he was living alone and Parkinsons had just been diagnosed. As he believed that the effects of this curse continued to linger, arrangements were made for him to see a *curandera*. The writers marvelled at the swiftness with which the elderly woman built rapport with Mr. Molina and moved the generally stoic man to tears of joy and she entered his world and concentrated her efforts on his complaint — the pain in his leg, which he said had plagued him since that fall many years ago. The *curandera* saw him for thirty minutes during which time she used holy water, prayer, touch, and the application of bee ointment to his pain. Interestingly, although Mr. Molina also viewed his Parkinson's as the result of a curse, he did not ask the healer to cure this problem.

Mr. Molina claimed relief for weeks afterward. The *curandera* stated that she would have to treat him at least three more times in order to effect a cure. However, before subsequent visits could be arranged, the elderly healer, who had congestive heart failure, said she was unable to provide further treatments, even though several people every day came to her house looking for help. The writer then located a *curandero* whose primary method was massage and who charged a flat fee, but Mr. Molina declined his services.

The therapist continues to read stories to the patient once a week, and although content still includes Mexican folklore, it also includes stories about the Mexican Revolution and translations into Spanish such as Hemingway's *Old Man and the Sea*. He remains without cognitive impairment and he attends twice daily kinesiotherapy and recreation therapy. His depression has not returned and at this writing his score on the Geriatric Depression Scale (Brink et al., 1982) was one (a score of zero to ten is normal, or no depression.)

Reports in the Literature on Curses

Treating a curse in non-elderly psychiatric patients has been reported on twice previously. Casper and Phillipus (1975) reported on fifteen cases of a curse, twelve of which improved through treatment with suggestion and antidepressant medication. Kreisman (1975) reported on the successful treatment of a curse that involved a *curandero*'s methods, although a *curandero* himself was not utilized.

General Assessment and Treatment Issues

As older adults of all ethnicities are especially sensitive to the stigma attached to mental health treatment, it is important for the therapist to accelerate the building of rapport, assessment and intervention. Before moving prematurely into personal and interpersonal issues, it is sometimes helpful for the therapist to utilize "exaggerated engagement" — deliberately exaggerating issues of time, interest and credibility — while attending to the multi-change process of problems and losses. (Gafner, 1987). With Mexican-American elders, the therapist needs to be especially attentive to issues of language, culture, religion, and belief system.

Assessing Level of Acculturation and Cultural Beliefs

In assessing one's level of acculturation, it might be helpful to ask clients if they identify with holidays such as the Day of the Dead or Cinco de Mayo. For the Spanish-speaking therapist, it is useful to ask clients if they prefer Spanish or English. Mr. Molina clearly preferred Spanish, while Mrs. Esquivel had a strong preference for English. Many clients will answer, "los dos," indicating that they are comfortable alternating between both languages. Also, the therapist needs to bear in mind that respect is especially important to Mexican-American elders.

In the authors' experience, the legend of La Llorona (Agogino et al., 1973), which dates from the Conquest, is nearly universally known among Mexican-Americans. To ask clients about La Llorona can help the therapist tap into cultural beliefs and build rapport. As children, Mexican-Americans are taught that the wind blowing at night is the sound of La Llorona looking for her lost child.

A Cautionary Note

Ramirez-Boulette (1980) noted that in all mental health settings Mexican-Americans need to be screened to rule out religious guilt and folk disorders. However, Trotter (1985) cautions health practitioners in general against analyzing folk disorders solely on sociocultural factors. Trotter, a medical anthropologist, notes that *susto* (fright), *empacho* (blocked intestine) and other presumably culture-bound syndromes might signal serious medical conditions, and that other times the conditions might be essentially harmless, but that their treatment, e.g., laundry bluing to treat *empacho*, could have significant medical consequences.

Using Folk Traditions and Beliefs in Treatment

Especially among nursing home residents like Mr. Molina, reminiscence (Zuniga, 1989) may be an integral part of treatment, and certainly an aspect of this treatment with Mexican-Americans can include rich and powerful recollections dealing with cultural beliefs and traditions. It is important to try understand their belief system, how they see the world and make sense out of it. Cultural beliefs are powerful and provide a sense of security, as well as connecting Mexican-American elders to their past. Rituals such as those performed by a *curandero* are empowered by the beliefs, which in turn empower the believer.

The writers often broach the subject of *curanderismo* with clients by gently inquiring with something like, "I've heard of people who have gotten better by going to a *curandero* . . . ." or "I wonder if spearmint tea would be good to take with your medication." This can lend an atmosphere of acceptance and permission to the session.

In closing, as we think about how we wish to introduce any possible strength or influence to bear on our clients' problems, the words of Prince (1981) come to mind: "A good healer of any culture is one who can provide relief from suffering."

For further reading:

Bless Me Ultima (1972). Anaya, R. Berkeley, CA: Tonatiuh International.
Mi Abuela Fumaba Puros/My Grandmother Smoked Cigars (1977). Ulibarri, S. Berkeley, CA: Quinto Sol.
The Serpent and the Rainbow (1985). Davis, W. N.Y., NY: Simon & Schuster.

REFERENCES

Agogino, G., Stevens, D. & Carlotta, L. (1973). Dona Marina and the legend of La Llorona. *Anthropological Journal of Canada*, 11 (1), 27-33.
Brink, T.L., Yesavage, J.A., Lum, O., Heersema, P., Adey, M. & Rose, T.L. (1982). Screening tests for geriatric depression. *Clinical Gerontologist*, 1 (1), 37-43.
Casper, E. & Phillipus, M. (1975). Fifteen cases of embrujada: Combining medication and suggestion in treatment. *Hospital Community Psychiatry*, 26 (5), 271-274.
Gafner, G. (1987). Engaging the elderly couple in marital therapy. *American Journal of Family Therapy*, 15 (4), 305-315.
Kiev, A. (1964). *Magic, Faith and Healing*. N.Y., NY: Free Press.
Kreisman, J. (1975). The curandero's apprentice. *American Journal of Psychiatry*, 32 (1), 81-83.
Marsh, W. & Hentges, K. (1988). Mexican folk remedies and conventional medical care. *American Family Physician*, 37, (3), 257-262.
Meredith, J. (1984). Ethnic medicine on the frontier. *Hispanic Journal of Behavioral Sciences*, 6 (3), 247-260.

Prince, R. (1981). The psychiatrist and folk healer. In Meyer, G. (Ed.) *Folk Medicine and Herbal Healing*. Springfield, Il: Charles C Thomas.

Ramirez-Boulette, T. (1980). Structured clinical interview model. Presentation at Advanced Clinical Symposium in Mental Health: El Paciente de Habla Hispana. La Jolla, CA: UCSD School of Medicine, June 13, 1980.

Romeo, L. (1990). Parallels between family therapy and *curanderismo*. Presentation at El Paso, TX: National Assn. of Social Workers Texas State Conference, Oct. 13, 1990.

Torres, E. (1983). *The Folk Healer: Mexican-American Tradition of Curanderismo*. Kingsville, TX: Nieves Press.

Trotter, R. (1985). Folk medicine in the southwest. *Postgraduate Medicine*, 78 (8), 167-179.

Zuniga, M. (1989). Mexican-American elderly and reminiscence: Interventions. *Journal of Gerontological Social Work*, 14 (3/4), 61-73.

SECTION FOUR:
SERVICE UTILIZATION

Chapter Eleven

The Self-Reliance Behavior of the Hispanic Elderly in Comparison to Their Use of Formal Mental Health Helping Networks

Richard Alton Starrett, PhD
Dan Rogers, MA
James T. Decker, PhD

Editor's Introduction

Starrett, Rogers, and Decker present survey data on the degree to which Hispanic aged use self-help, informal networks, and institutional assistance. The main finding was that self-help was the principal resource. Unfortunately, there is no evidence that such self-help was effective in nurturing mental health.

One previous issue of *Clinical Gerontologist* looked at self-help in the nursing home:

1990 IX (3,4) 92, 103, 148, 152, 163, 172, 177, 185, 186

Richard Alton Starrett, Dan Rogers, and James T. Decker are affiliated with the California School of Professional Psychology, Fresno.

In memory of my father, Alton B. Starrett (1905-1990).

The authors would like to express their gratitude to Carmela Lacayo, President of the National Association of Hispanic Elderly, for providing the data for this study.

and the use of self-monitoring and self-management has been discussed by several articles and clinical comments:

1983 I (3) 45-52
1985 IV (1) 72-73
1985 IV (2) 38-40, 48-51
1989 VIII (4) 3-11, 43-45

Empirical studies of the mental health utilization behavior of the elderly are relatively absent from the gerontological literature (Coulton & Frost, 1982). Only one study exists that attempts to predict why the Hispanic elderly use formal mental health services (Starrett, Decker, Walters, & Araujo, 1989). Most of the research on the use of Hispanic mental health services is of a descriptive nature and none use conceptual frameworks to analyze the complexities of the utilization process (Baron, 1981; Newton, 1980, 1981; Padilla & Lindholm, 1983; Rogler et al., 1983).

None of the current research employs Anderson and Newman's (1973) service utilization framework to compare the characteristics of the Hispanic elderly users of formal mental health services (i.e., use of professionals, doctors or the church) to non-users (self-reliant) of services.

There is no literature that attempts to compare the characteristics of Hispanic elderly who use mental health services to non-users. In a review of help-seeking behavior in general Gourash (1978) suggested that *nonusers* differ by age, race and social class. Auslander and Lutwin (1990), in a recent study of 200 elderly applicants and non-applicants for social services found that non-applicants were younger, married, had low functional disabilities and physical capacity, and had a greater size of informal network (i.e., more friends, children and neighbors). However, the main assumption in the literature is that the majority of people with mental health problems seek out help first from their informal support and, as a last resort, turn to formal help. What about the elderly who are only dependent on their own self-reliance for help?

CONCEPTUAL FRAMEWORK

A sophisticated classification system was proposed by Andersen and Newman (1973) and later suggested by Ward (1977) for studying health and social service use among the elderly. This model was employed by Coulto and Frost (1982) as a utilization of mental health framework and subsequently tested by them. Moreover, the utilization behaviors of the

African American, Hispanic, Mexican American, Puerto Rican, and Cuban elderly have all substantiated this model as adequate for minority elderly populations (Starrett, Decker, Walters, & Araujo, 1989; Starrett, Mindel, & Wright, 1983, 1984). This model was utilized by the current authors to conceptualize the individual's demand for mental health services as a linear function of a complex pattern of relationships among Predisposing, Enabling, and Need Factors. The model suggests that some elderly are more predisposed to use services, based on certain background characteristics, such as demographic, social structural, and beliefs (Predisposing factor). Although individuals may have differential propensities to use services, the use of services is contingent upon the availability and accessibility of community and family resources (Enabling factor). Finally, assuming that the above conditions exist, the individual must recognize the presence of a need for services and be motivated to take some form of action before actual service use takes place (Need factor).

Recent research on the utilization of social services by the elderly has found support for the importance of the Predisposing and Enabling factors in the use of services. The predisposing variables that were found significantly related to use were living arrangements, education, not married, ethnicity, Hispanicism, years at residence, age, citizenship, language difficulty, number of children, and gender (Escobar & Kartines, 1983; Krout, 1983; McCaslin, 1989; Starrett, 1989a, 1989b; Starrett & Decker, 1984, 1987; Starrett, Decker, Araujo, & Walters, 1988; Starrett, Mindel, & Wright, 1983, 1984; Starrett, Wright, & Mindel, 1988; Wan & O'Dell, 1981). The enabling variables that were found to predict use were availability of service, knowledge, transportation, contact with children, income, age density, contact with friends, and church attendance (Escobar & Kartines, 1983; Krout, 1983; McCaslin, 1989; Mindel & Wright, 1981; Starrett, Decker et al., 1988; Starrett, Mindel, & Wright, 1983, 1984; Starrett, Wright, & Mindel, 1988; Wan & O'Dell, 1981). The need variables found to determine use were number of social service needs, health, and ADL (Escobar & Kartines, 1983; Krout, 1983; McCaslin, 1989; Mindel & Wright, 1981; Starrett, 1989a, 1989b; Starrett & Decker, 1984, 1987; Starrett, Decker et al., 1988; Starrett, Mindel, & Wright, 1983, 1984; Starrett, Wright, & Mindel, 1988; Wan & O'Dell, 1981).

The use of social service appears to reflect a different pattern of use than medical service use. Knowledge of social services was the best predictor of use by the Hispanic elderly (Starrett, 1989b), Mexican American and Puerto Rican elderly (Starrett & Decker, 1984; Starrett, Decker et al.,

1988; Starrett, Mindel & Wright, 1983, 1984), and the general population (Krout, 1983). However, several researchers found need to be the best predictor of use among the white and black elderly population (McCaslin, 1989; Mindel & Wright, 1981; Wan & O'Dell, 1981) and Puerto Rican population (Starrett, Decker et al., 1988). Moreover all these researchers found the other Enabling and the Predisposing factors to have both directly and indirectly affected use. The varieties within social service use appear to reflect the more discretionary nature of social versus medical services, as suggested by Ward (1977). One important exception to the above research was a study of the Cuban elderly by Escobar and Kartines (1983) that found Hispanicism (i.e., cultural identity) to be the best predictor of social service use, followed by health and years of residence. The differences found in this study may be due to measurement issues, i.e., the dependent variable was a combination of all types of formal services, inadequate measures of need, and no measure of knowledge or other relevant enabling/predisposing variables.

The purpose of the present study was to develop and evaluate a model of formal mental health utilization behavior by the Hispanic elderly compared to self-reliance behavior. More specifically, the study investigated which factors (Predisposing, Enabling, Need) are the strongest determinants of use of a professional for mental health problems, which factors (Predisposing, Enabling, Need) are the strongest determinants of use of a physician for mental health problems, which factors (Predisposing, Enabling, Need) are the strongest determinants of use of a church for mental health problems, and which factors (Predisposing, Enabling, Need) are the strongest determinants of self-reliance.

METHODS

Sample

The data analyzed in this study were from a data set that was collected in 1979-1980 entitled "A National Study to Assess the Service Needs of the Hispanic Elderly" (principal investigator, Carmela G. Lacayo, 1980). The data were provided by the National Association for Hispanic Elderly and were gathered from a national probability sample of 1,805 noninstitutionalized Hispanic individuals age 55 and over.

A multistage probability sampling procedure, with geographic stratification introduced in the first stage, was employed to randomly select elderly Hispanic respondents. Geographic stratification by region was chosen to assure adequate representation of Hispanics in regions with the highest density of Hispanics. The final sample represented 15 states, with California, Texas, Florida, and New York having a heavier sampling of elderly Hispanics. It was estimated that the sampling error was approximately 5%.

The characteristics of the sample were as follows: ethnic identity — Mexican American 59.3%, Puerto Rican 15.8%, Cuban 6.2%, other Hispanic 18.8%; sexual composition — 48.6% males and 51.4% females; mean age — 65.5 years; marital status — not married 47%, married 53%; mean education — 5 years; mean income $3,000.00; mental health problems — 8% used priest, 5% used doctor, 2% used agency, 1% used a counselor or psychologist, 83% did not utilize any service; in contrast, 13% had family problems, 40% were depressed, 43% had worries and 21.9% had fears.

This study employs Andersen and Newman's (1973) framework to classify and analyze the 31 variables conceptualized as determinants of mental health use behavior and self-reliance behavior by the Hispanic elderly.

Measurement

Data were obtained from interviews administered in the respondent's home, using a pretested instrument constructed by the National Association for Hispanic Elderly in consultation with the Administration on Aging, the U.S. Census Bureau, and Kaiser Permanente's Research Department. The final instrument was a combination of Older American's Resource and Service Functional Assessment Questionnaire (OARS), and the Subjective Distress Scale of Psychiatric Status Schedule (PSS). The modified PSS included items that measured how many Hispanic elderly had experienced mental health problems in the last 6 months in the following areas: depression, family problems, worry, and fear. The instrument was translated into Spanish and administered by bilingual interviewers.

Thirty variables were selected for this study and classified by Andersen and Newman's (1973) framework as either Predisposing, Enabling, or Need or Use Factors.

The utilization of mental health services was measured by summing which service (i.e., professional, physician, or church) each individual used when he or she was depressed, worried, afraid, or had a family problem. The scale for using a professional (i.e., counselor, psychologist, or an agency), the church, or a physician for mental health problems was measured by summing the number of times each service provider was utilized for each problem area (i.e., depression, family problems, worry,

and fear) by the Hispanic elderly. The scale for self-reliance was measured by summing the number of times each individual used no one when
he or she were depressed, had family problems, worries or fears.

Data Analysis

The method of analysis employed to test and compare the use of formal
mental health utilization behavior to self-reliant behavior was that of block
hierarchical regression analysis. Each block of variables (need, family,
community, and predisposing) is run sequentially against each dependent
variable. The results of the analysis give us the ability to determine which
of the four types of mental health behavior (i.e., using a professional,
physician, church) and self-reliance explain the most variance, which determinants are the most important in explaining the utilization of mental
health service and self reliant behavior, and what are the common and
unique differences across service types.

RESULTS

The zero order correlation coefficients, means, and standard deviations
for all the variables, related to the four criterion variables: use of a professional, physician, the church, and self-reliance, were analyzed. The
results suggest that the model was strongest in predicting self-reliance for
mental health problems, with 36% of the variance accounted for, followed
by use of the church accounting for 17%, use of physician with 9%, and
use of a professional 8% of the variance.

The results for reliance on self to solve mental health problems by the
Hispanic Elderly indicate that 11 of the 31 independent variables employed in the study directly affected use of self. The Need factor accounted for most of the variance (33.26%) followed by the Enabling factor (2.42%) and Predisposing factor (.14%). With respect to the Need
factor, depression (.52%), family problems (.22%), fear (− .05%), worry
(− .05%) and functional ability (.10%) directly affected self-reliance behavior. *Those Hispanic elderly who were more depressed, had more family problems, had greater functional ability, were less worried or afraid
depended upon themselves exclusively to solve their problems.* Of the Enabling factor, six variables, contact with friends (− .06%), participating
in senior church activities (− .06%), church attendance (− .06%), residential stability (.04%) age density (.08) and living with grandchildren
(.04) directly affected nonuse of services. *Those elderly who had less*

contact with friends, participated in senior church activities less, attended church less, were less stable residentially, were in a higher age density area, and lived with grandchildren were more self-reliant. Those elderly who were housewives (.04%) were more predisposed to be self-reliant.

The major finding of this study was that the Hispanic elderly rely on themselves to solve their mental health problem more often than they use the church, physician, or professional. This finding holds true across service type despite the fact that Hispanic elderly who depend on themselves for help were more depressed and had more family problems than the other service types. These results can be interpreted to mean either that self-reliance behavior is a normal coping mechanism or that alternative mechanisms are not employed because of family or institutional barriers (Padilla & Lindholm, 1983; Padilla & Ruiz, 1973). This finding raises the question: Is self-reliance an adaptive or maladaptive coping mechanism? Only future research can answer this question.

In the current study, need was the strongest predictor of use, thus seeking mental health help is more like health utilization than social service utilization by the Hispanic elderly. It appears that *being depressed, followed by having family problems, are the strongest motivators for seeking help across service type*. However, the pattern of service use varied considerably across service type, with depression and family problems being more important determinants in self-reliant behavior.

In comparing the differences in use of the church, physicians, professionals, and self-reliant behavior across groups, having lower functional ability directly affected use of a physician and was not important to the other groups. Thus, in addition to depression and having family problems, a secondary indicator for use of the physician for mental health problems is poorer health. This, however, may be the presenting problem to the primary care physician which has led several studies to emphasize the need for additional mental health training for physicians and the need for emphasis of appropriate referrals (Comstock & Schrager, 1979; Schurman, Kramer & Mitchell, 1985; Waxman & Corner, 1984).

The Enabling factor was the strongest predictor of the use of the church for mental health problems, followed by self-reliance behavior, use of the church, use of physician, and use of professionals. Church utilization was uniquely predicted by church attendance, participation in senior activities, high neighborhood cohesiveness, and fewer elderly living in the area. It seems logical to assume that church use will be greater for those elderly with greater contact with the church and who live in more cohesive neighborhoods. It also seems that elders who live in more heterogeneous neighborhoods seek out service more from the church. It may be that contact with younger neighbors facilitates this process by increased interaction with the younger generation and sharing of knowledge.

Since the Hispanic elderly used the church twice as much as any other formal source, mental health outreach efforts should focus on networking with churches and church groups in addition to training of clergy and providing referral information. This may be of particular importance to those Hispanic elderly living in poorer sections of the city with higher density of elderly (Bruman, 1987; Keefe, Padilla, & Carlos, 1979; Steinitz, 1982; Szapocznik, Lasaga, & Perry, 1979; Taylor & Chatters, 1986).

The factors that enable self-reliant behavior are quite different from the other service types with the Hispanic elderly who have less contact with friends, less church contact, less stable residentially, live in higher age density areas and with their grandchildren solving their own mental health problems. This pattern appears quite opposite of what we would expect if self-reliant behavior is an effective coping mechanism. This seems to be a picture of an isolated inner city Hispanic elderly except for the fact that they are living with grandchildren which might facilitate their coping behaviors. This enigma begs for future research.

The pattern of service use for the physician and professional within the Enabling factor is quite different than for the use of the church. The Hispanic elderly use both service types because they have been living in the area longer, thus facilitating their use of a physician or professional. Living arrangements are also important for use of both service types. It appears that living with a relative or parents facilitates use of professionals and that living with sibling or with spouse facilitates use of a physician. These results have important outreach implications. Moreover, lack of contact with relatives encourages use of professionals. This may suggest that more independent or isolated Hispanics tend to use professionals. Last, living in an urban area facilitates use of a physician rather than other types of services (Bruman, 1987; Keefe et al., 1979). This may be due to greater accessibility, availability, and number of physicians in urban areas.

Regarding the Predisposing factor, more variability is seen across service type than within the other factors. Only nativity is important for both the use of professionals and physicians. Those Hispanic elderly who use professionals are uniquely characterized as being born in the U.S., better educated, and perceiving more sex discrimination. These results suggest that acculturation leads to greater use of a professional (Cervantes & Castro, 1985). The Hispanics who use a physician are born outside the U.S. and of Cuban descent. This seems to suggest that in more traditional cultures outside the U.S., the physician is a common source of help for psychological distress, and this pattern continues after emigration to the U.S. (Karno & Edgerton, 1969). However, it must be kept in mind that most Hispanic elderly do not use either professionals (8%) or physicians (9%) more than the church (17%). These results are supported by an early study by Keefe et al. (1979) that found similar results. The variables that predispose the Hispanic elderly to use the church for mental health problems are being a female, non-Catholic, and retired. These results suggest that contact with the church facilitates help seeking for all groups; however, this is especially important for the non-Catholic population. The only variable that predisposed the Hispanic elderly to be self-reliant was being a housewife. It may well be that by being at home and more isolated, with limited social contacts, that those women who work encourage more self-reliant behavior. These findings have important outreach, service delivery, and policy implications.

This study raises a provocative question: When an elderly individual is depressed or has family problems, is self-reliant behavior an effective coping mechanism or an indication of lack of alternatives or barriers to use? Moreover, having a mental health problem was more indicative of self-reliant behavior than use of formal mental health network (church, physicians, professions). It is also clear that within the formal mental health network the Hispanic elderly prefer using the church over the physicians or other professionals (Casas & Keefe, 1978; Cervantes & Castro, 1985; Newton, 1980).

REFERENCES

Aday, L., & Eichorn, R. (1972). *The utilization of health services: Indices and correlates*. National Center for Health Services Research and Development, DHEW Publication No. (HSM) 73-3003. Washington, DC: U.S. Government Printing Office.

Andersen, R., & Aday, L.A. (1978). Access of medical care in the U.S.: Realized and potential. *Medical Care, 16*, 533-546.

Andersen, R., McGreely, R., Kravits, J., & Anderson, O.W. (1972). *Health services use national trends and variations, 1953-1971*. DHEW Publication No. (HSM) 73-3004. Washington, DC: U.S. Government Printing Office.

Andersen, R., & Newman, J.F. (1973). Societal and individual determinants of medical care utilization in the United States. *Milbank Memorial Fund Quarterly, 51*, 95-124.

Auslander, G.K. & Litwin, H. (1990). Social support networks and formal help seeking: Differences between applicants to social services and a nonapplicant sample. *Journal of Gerontology, 45,* (3), 5112-5119.

Baron, A. (1981). *Explanations in Chicano psychology.* New York: Praeger.

Barrera, M. Jr. (1978). Mexican-American mental health service utilization: A critical examination of some proposed variables. *Community Mental Health Journal, 14* (1), 35-45.

Blau, S.Z., Oser, G.T., & Stephens, R.C. (1979). Aging, social class and ethnicity. *Pacific Sociological Review, 22,* 501-525.

Bruman, L. (1987). Race differences in professional help seeking. *American Journal of Community Psychology, 15,* 473-489.

Cantor, M. (1985). Lifespace and the social support of the inner city elderly at New York. *The Gerontologist, 15,* 23-26.

Casas, S., & Keefe, S. (1978). *Family and mental health in the Mexican American community.* Los Angeles: UCLA Spanish Speaking Mental Health Resource Center.

Cervantes, R.C., & Castro, F.G. (1985). Stress, coping and Mexican-American mental health: A systematic review. *Hispanic Journal of Behavior Sciences,* 7(1), 1-73.

Comstock, D., & Schrager, L. (1979). Hospital services and community characteristics: The physician as mediator. *Journal of Health and Social Behavior, 20,* 59-97.

Coulton, C., & Frost, C. (1982). Use of social and health services by the elderly. *Journal of Health and Social Behavior, 23,* 330-339.

Cutler, S. (1975). Transportation and changes in life satisfaction. *The Gerontologist, 15,* 155-159.

Downing, R. (1977). The older person in crisis: An exploratory study of 250 older persons. *The Gerontologist, 17*(5), 28-29.

Escobar, L., & Kartines, M. (1983). Psychosocial predictors of service utilization among Cuban elderly. *Journal of Community Psychology, 11,* 355-362.

Gourish, N. (1978). Help-seeking: A review of the literature. *American Journal of Community Psychology, 6* (5), 413-423.

Harris, L., & Associates. (1975). *The myth and reality of aging in America.* Washington, DC: National Council on Aging.Hershey, J.C., Luft, H.S. & Glanaris, J. (1975). Making sense out of utilization data. *Medical Care, 13,* 838-854.

Karno, M., & Edgerton, R.B. (1969). Perceptions of mental illness in a Mexican American community. *Archives of General Psychiatry, 20,* 233-238.

Keefe, S.E., Padilla, A.M. & Carlos, M.L. (1979). The Mexican American extended family as an emotional support system. *Human Organization, 38,* 144-152.

Krout, J.A. (1983). Utilization of services by the elderly. *Social Service Review, 58,* 281-290.

Lacayo, C.G. (1980). *A national study to assess the service needs of the Hispanic elderly*. Washington, DC: Department of Health and Human Services, Library of Congress, No. 81-66632.

Larson, R. (1978). Thirty years of research on the subjective well-being of older Americans. *Journal of Gerontology, 33*, 109-125.

Lawton, M.P. (1983). Environment and other determinants of well-being in older people. *The Gerontologist, 23*, 349-357.

Lopez-Aqueres, W., Kemp, B., Staples, F., & Brummel-Smith, L. (1984). Use of health services by older Hispanics. *Journal of American Geriatric Society, 32*, 435-440.

Lowry, L. (1979). *Social work with the aging*. New York: Harper & Row.

McCaslin, R. (1989). A new look at service utilization. *Journal of Gerontological Social Work, 14*, 16-30.

McKinlay, J.B. (1972). Some approaches and problems in the study of the use of services – An overview. *Journal of Health and Social Behavior, 13*, 369-382.

Mindel, C.H., & Wright, R., Jr. (1981). The use of social services by black and white elderly: The role of social support systems. *Journal of Gerontological Social Work, 4*, 107-120.

Mutran, E., & Ferrano, K. (1988). Medical need and use of services among older men and women. *Journal of Gerontology, 43*, 3162-3171.

Neugarten B. (1974). Age groups in American society and the use of the young-old. *Annals of American Academy of Political and Social Science, 415*, 187-198.

Newton, F.C. (1980). Issues in research and service delivery among Mexican American elderly: A concise statement with recommendations. *The Gerontologist, 2*, 208-213.

Newton, F.C. (1981). The Hispanic elderly: A review of health, social and psychological factors. In A. Baron (Ed.), *Explanations in Chicano Psychology* (pp. 68-102). New York: Praeger.

Padilla, A.M., & Lindholm, L.S. (1983). *Hispanic Americans' future behavioral science research directives* (Occasional Paper No. 17). Los Angeles: University of California, Spanish Speaking Mental Health Research Center.

Padilla, A.M., & Ruiz, R.A. (1973). *Latino mental health: A review of the literature*, DHEW Publication No. (HSM) 73-9143. Washington, DC: U.S. Government Printing Office.

Ralston, P.A., & Griggs, M.B. (1980). Factors affecting participation in sewing center: Race, sex and socioeconomic differences. *Journal of Minority Aging, 5*, 209-217.

Rogler, L.H., Cooney, R.S., Constantino, G., Early, B.F., Grossman, B., Gurek, D.T., Malgady, R., & Rodriguez, O. (1983). *A conceptual framework for mental health research on Hispanic populations* (Monograph No. 10). Bronx, NY: Fordham University, Hispanic Research Center.

Schurman, R., Kramer, P., Mitchell, S. (1985). The hidden mental health network. *Archives of General Psychiatry, 42*, 89-94.

Shanas, E. (1979). The family as a social support system in old age. *The Gerontologist, 19,* 169-174.

Starrett, R. (1989a). A comparison of the social service utilization behavior of the Cuban and Puerto Rican elderly. *Hispanic Journal of Behavioral Sciences, 2,* 341-353.

Starrett, R. (1989b). The role of environmental awareness and support networks in Hispanic elderly's use of social services. *Journal of Community Psychology, 3,* 259-273.

Starrett, R.A., & Decker, J.T. (1984). The use of discretionary services by the Hispanic elderly. *California Sociologist, 7,* 159-180.

Starrett, R.A., & Decker, J.T. (1987). The utilization of social services by the Mexican American elderly. In R. Dobroff (Ed.), *Ethnicity and gerontological social work* (pp. 87-102). New York: The Haworth Press, Inc.

Starrett, R., Decker, J., Araujo, A., & Walters, G. (1988). The social service utilization of the Puerto Rican elderly. *Aging and Society, 7,* 445-458.

Starrett, R., Decker, J., Walters, G., & Araujo, A. (1989). The Cuban elderly and their service use. *Journal of Applied Gerontology, 3,* 69-85.

Starrett, R.A., Mindel, C.H., & Wright, R. (1983). Influence of support systems on the use of social services by the Hispanic elderly. *Social Work Research and Abstracts, 19*(3), 35-40.

Starrett, R.A., Mindel, C.H., & Wright, R. (1984). Influence of support systems or the use of social services by the Hispanic elderly. In J. Hopps & T. Tripud (Eds.), *People of color* (pp. 35-40). New York: NASW.

Starrett, R., Wright, R., Jr., & Mindel, C. (1988). The use of social services by Hispanics: A comparison of Mexican American, Puerto Rican, and Cuban elderly. *Journal of Social Service Research, 11,* 459-489.

Steinitz, L. (1982). The local church as support for the elderly. *Journal of Gerontological Social Work, 4*(27), 43-53.

Szapocznic, J., Lasaga, S.H., & Perry, P. (1979). Outreach in the delivery of mental health services to Hispanic elderly. *Hispanic Journal of Behavioral Sciences, 1*(1), 21-40.

Taylor, R., & Chatters, L.M. (1986). Church based informal support among elderly black. *Gerontologist, 26,* 637-642.

Wan, T.T., & O'Dell, B. (1981). Factors affecting use of social and health services among the elderly. *Aging and Society, 1,* 55-115.

Wan, T.T., & Soifer, S.S. (1974). Determinants of physician utilization: A causal analysis. *Journal of Health and Social Behavior, 15,* 100-108.

Ward, R.A. (1977). Services for older people: An integrated framework for research. *Journal of Health and Social Behavior, 18,* 61-70.

Waxman, H., & Corner, E. (1984). Physicians' recognition, diagnosis and treatment of mental disorders in elderly medical patients. *The Gerontologist, 24,* 593-597.

Wolinsky, P.S. (1978). Assessing the effects of predisposing, enabling, and illness-morbidity characteristics on health service utilization. *Journal of Health and Social Behavior, 19,* 384-396.

Wolinsky, P.D., & Cole, R.M. (1984). Physician and hospital utilization among noninstitutionalized elderly: An analysis of the health and interview survey. *Journal of Gerontology, 39,* 334-341.

Wright, R., Creecy, R.F., & Brog, W.E. (1979). The black elderly and their use of health care services: A causal analysis. *Journal of Gerontological Social Work, 2,* 11-28.

Chapter Twelve

Barriers to Health Care Access Faced by Elderly Mexican Americans

Ernesto O. Parra, MD, MPH
David V. Espino, MD

Editor's Introduction

Parra and Espino describe specific barriers that elder Hispanics face in getting mental health care and connecting with other useful formal networks and institutions. Policy recommendations are given.

Two previous issues of *Clinical Gerontologist* have contained articles on the topic of mental health care delivery:

1986 V 1-18
1987 VI (4) 3-14

OVERVIEW OF ACCESS PROBLEM

Most Mexican American senior citizens find that they are faced with financial and institutional barriers when they try to obtain medical attention in the United States. Additionally, they have unique needs that must be met before they can effectively access and utilize health care services. This article will review the various types of health access problems that older Mexican Americans struggle with and recommend ways of alleviating them.

Ernesto O. Parra is Assistant Professor, Department of Family Practice and David V. Espino is Assistant Professor, Division of Geriatrics, Department of Family Practice, both at the University of Texas Health Science Center, San Antonio.

It is important for physicians, administrators, and other health providers to be aware of these barriers and needs. Such professionals can direct future changes in the health care system that would result in the improved health status of elderly Mexican Americans.

FINANCIAL BARRIERS

Several studies have already identified that the strongest predictor of poor health and access to health care among Hispanics is the lack of health insurance (Munoz, 1988; Hubbell, 1989; Freeman, 1990). Approximately, 30% of Hispanics have no private health insurance, Medicaid or Medicare coverage compared to 11% of the general population (USHHS, 1986). Among the Hispanic elderly, an estimated 19% are not covered by any type of health insurance program, including medicare and medicaid, compared to 4% of White elderly. The lack of health insurance is associated with poor health and low income (Lopez, 1984; Churchill, 1987). Among elderly Hispanics, nearly 47% are below or at the near poverty level compared to 25% of the White elderly (Maldonado, 1988). The large proportion of poor elderly Mexican Americans without private health insurance places this ethnic subgroup at high risk for not receiving any health maintenance care or urgent medical attention. On one hand, they may not meet their state's strict criteria for poverty, and be ineligible for Medicaid. On the other hand, they may not be able to pay Medicare's Part B supplemental premiums for outpatient physician visits (Estes, 1986).

Lack of private or government health insurance, and limited financial resources among aged Mexican Americans prevents their utilization of health care. Out-of-pocket expenses for hospitalization, outpatient clinic visits, and prescription medications deter elderly individuals from receiving adequate medical care. Those who are covered by third-party payers are often hampered from obtaining care because of the high costs of deductibles for hospital admission and co-payments for outpatient visits. Furthermore, certain third-party payers will not reimburse particular medical services or equipment that is crucial to elderly individuals, such as mental health, dental care, home nursing assistance, podiatric care, screening exams, hearing aids, eyeglasses, and special laboratory or radiological testing (ACOP 1984).

Ultimately, the fate of most elderly Mexican Americans who seek medical care is to use state government and county health facilities. Unfortunately, such facilities are usually too understaffed and under funded to provide prompt, adequate, and specialized care to older individuals.

Health professionals may help lessen the financial barriers to health care for older Mexican Americans by advocating to the state and federal government that the elderly not be left without some type of health insurance. This may be partially accomplished by:

1. Advocating federal, state, and county governments to adopt cost effective financing strategies to insure the elderly and to prevent the continual steep rise in catastrophic health care costs,
2. Encouraging the use of bilingual educational programs that assist employees in understanding eligibility requirements for Medicare and how to use it,
3. Promoting the use of bilingual social service assistance to elderly individuals to help them enroll in Medicaid,
4. Urging that state legislation be modified to raise the income level that the state defines as poverty so that more elderly individuals could participate in Medicaid and receive such care,
5. Identifying those examinations and screening tests, such as mammography, that should be covered by Medicare as necessary preventative care measures.

INSTITUTIONAL BARRIERS

The growing number of elderly individuals have placed an increased demand for nursing home accommodations. Yet, even though older Hispanics represent greater than 2% of the U.S. aged population, they compose less than 1% of elderly in nursing homes (Watson, 1986). The primary reasons why Hispanics under utilize nursing homes can be attributed to racial discrimination, high cost, insensitivity to cultural customs, and communication problems that occur in among these institutions. Nursing homes in the U.S. have traditionally been staffed by administrators and caretakers who only speak English. Such staff may alienate Hispanic elderly and their families. Similar problems play a role in the under use of hospitals and clinics by elderly Hispanics.

In general, hospitals and outpatient health care facilities that serve a significant number of Mexican American patients do not adequately address the cultural and language obstacles that face their patients. Recent studies of elderly utilization of community health and mental health clinics, where cost for care was not a factor, suggest that differences in use by an ethnic group are associated with programmatic differences (Light, 1986; Scheffler, 1989). Services such as, bilingual caretakers, Hispanic counselors and case managers would greatly benefit Mexican American geriatric patients and the families that care for them. Unfortunately, the incentives behind the reimbursement policies for hospitalization by Medicare (DRGs) and for nursing home care and outpatient care by Medicaid are for these institutions to provide less services (Ostrander, 1985; Culpepper, 1986). The medical care received by the aged is significantly limited and fragmented by these policies.

The location of a hospital, clinic, or pharmacy may yield it inaccessible to older Mexican Americans (Cromley, 1986; Shannon, 1985). Those inpatient or ambulatory facilities that are not geographically strategic within the Hispanic community to allow easy access by elderly residents and their families, will not be utilized by these individuals. Additionally, inadequate planning and resources to meet the transportation needs of the older Hispanics will render such facilities ineffective (Cluff, 1983).

Recommendations to health professionals that seek to reduce the institutional barriers to health care for older Mexican Americans include:

1. Incorporating elderly Mexican American residents into the facility's board of directors to help ensure that culturally sensitive and appealing services are offered to the geriatric community,
2. Advocating government officials to support initiatives for long term care management that bridge the gaps between inpatient, ambulatory, and home care assistance to aged Mexican Americans and their families.
3. Advising city planners of strategic geographic sites for programs aimed at reaching the geriatric Hispanic population,
4. Recruiting bilingual health care providers to work at facilities which service the Hispanic elderly,
5. Educating health care personnel about the needs of their geriatric patients and clients, and
6. Providing minibus service, travel vouchers, or home health aid to older residents that have difficulty obtaining transportation assistance to their health facility.

SPECIAL NEEDS

In order to make head way at improving health care delivery to geriatric Mexican Americans, it is necessary for health providers to appreciate some fundamental characteristics of this group.

A large proportion of older Mexican Americans are functionally illiterate in English. Many had worked when they were children to help support their family, leaving them little opportunity to obtain a formal education. Consequently, many may have difficulty understanding the verbal recommendations by physicians and nurses as well as following the written directions on prescriptions. Creative educational methods and materials are needed to empower older Hispanics about how they can improve their health status.

Traditional folk remedies and health beliefs play an influential role in the health maintenance of elder Mexican Americans (Marsh, 1988). For these individuals the use of herbs, culturally specific home remedies, and faith healers (curanderos), may still be regarded as primary forms of care for persons who suffer from physical or mental ailments (Kreisman, 1975). It is essential that health professionals caring for such elders understand the cultural concepts behind the healing process and the use of traditional remedies (Ripley 1986, Reinert 1986). This may give professionals the skill to effectively integrate Western medicine into the health belief model of their patients and improve their compliance with current medical therapies (Chesney, 1980).

Finally, it is crucial that counseling and supportive services be provided for family members who care for senior Mexican Americans. The increased reliance on family for an older member's care may place an economic and social strain on Hispanic families attempting to improve their socioeconomic status (Gratton, 1988). Such a strain may lead to a deterioration in the family dynamics that supports the elder's health. It is advantageous for the health of elders to supply their guardians with the necessary information and assistance that will result in the family's participation with the health care plan. Mexican American families may be particularly receptive to this approach since they have traditionally assumed responsibility for the complete care of their aged members.

Proposals for addressing the special needs of Mexican American elderly include:

1. The development of educational methods and materials on geriatric health care information that can be understood by older individuals who may have a small amount of formal education and use Spanish as their first language,
2. The employment of culturally sensitive outreach programs using flyers, community newspapers, and local radio and television networks to inform elders on proper health maintenance and health facilities that are available to assist them,
3. The participation of health care staff in programs where they can learn to address the peculiarities of treating older Mexican Americans regarding their literacy, family support, and alternative cultural remedies they use,

4. The establishment of a family assistance program in the clinic setting for family members who could benefit from counseling, education, and social support services involved in caring for an aged person,

5. The enrollment of elderly individuals into existing community based elderly programs such as activity centers, nutrition centers, and Meals on Wheels.

SUMMARY

There are three general areas that need attention in order to improve the health care of older Mexican Americans. The first is lessening the financial burden of the elderly who are sick or who need health care maintenance. The second requires the modification of hospital, clinic, and nursing home policies to prevent discrimination and to facilitate their use by elder Hispanics. Finally, the development of community based, culturally sensitive health facilities that provide outreach programs for the aged and assistance for their families.

REFERENCES

Chesney AP, Thompson BL, et al. Mexican-American folk medicine: implications for the family physician. J Fam Prac. 1980; 11(4): 567-74.

Churchill LR. Health care, social justice and the elderly. No Carolina Med J. 1987; 48(11): 587.

Cluff LE. Problems of the health-impaired elderly: A foundation's experience in geriatrics. J Am Geriatr Soc. 1983; 31(11): 665-72.

Cromley EK, Shannon GW. Locating ambulatory medical care facilities for the elderly. Health Serv Res. 1986; 21(4): 499-514.

Culpepper S, Murphy J, Fretweel M. Biology, primary care, family, and community. A basis for rational geriatric care. Clin Geriatric Med. 1986; 2(1): 37-51.

Espino DV, Medication usage in elderly Hispanic: What we know and what we need to know. Proceedings on improving drug use among Hispanic elders. Nat Hisp Counc Aging. Washington D.C., 1988. pp 7-11.

Estes CL, The aging enterprise: In whose interests? Int J Health Services. 1986; 16(2): 243-51.

Freeman HE, Aiken LH et al. Uninsured working-age adults: Characteristics and consequences. Health Serv Res. 1990; 24(6): 811-23.

Gratton B, Wilson V. Family support systems and the minority elderly: A cautionary analysis. J Geront Soc Work. 1988; 13(1/2): 81-93.

Hubbell F, Waitzkin H et al. Evaluating health-care needs of the poor: A community-oriented approach. Am J Med. 1989; 87(2): 127-31.

Kreisman JJ. The curandero's apprentice: A therapeutic integration of folk and medical healing. Am J Psych. 1975; 132(1): 81-3.

Light E, Lebowitz BD, Baily F. CMHC's and elderly services: An analysis of direct service and indirect service delivery sites. Comm Ment Health J. 1986; 22(4): 294-302.

Long-term care of the elderly. Health and public policy committee, American College of Physicians. Ann Inter Med 1984; 100(5): 760-3.

Lopez AW, Kemp B, et al. Health needs of the Hispanic elderly. J Am Geriatric Soc. 1984; 32(3): 191-8.

Maldonado D. The Hispanic elderly: Vulnerability in old age. South Methodist University. 1988, Draft.

Marsh WW, Hentges K. Mexican folk remedies and conventional medical care. Am Fam Prac. 1988; 37(3): 257-262.

Munoz E. Care for the Hispanic poor: A growing segment of American society. JAMA. 1988; 260(18): 2711-2.

Ostrander V. Medicare DRGs pose problems for elderly. Hospitals. 1985; 56(24): 75-6.

Report of the secretary's task force on black and minority health: Hispanic health issues. U.S. Dept of Health and Human Services. 1986; 8:11-42.

Reinert BR. The health care beliefs and values of Mexican-Americans. Home Health Care Nur. 1986; 4(5): 23-31.

Ripley GD. Mexican-American folk remedies: Their place in health care. Texas Med. 1986; 82:41-44.

Scheffler RM, Miller AB. Demand analysis of mental health service use among ethnic subpopulations. Inquiry. 1989; 26(2): 202-15.

Shannon GW, Cromley EK, Fink JL. Pharmacy patronage among the elderly: selected racial and geographical patterns. Soc Sci Med. 1985; 20(1): 85-93.

Watson W. Nursing homes and the mental health of minority residents: some problems and needed research. U.S. Department of Health and Human Services. Alcohol, Drug Abuse, and Mental Health Administration. Monograph: Mental illness in nursing homes: Agenda for research. 1986. pp. 267-79.

Chapter Thirteen

Mexican-American Involuntary Arrival at Crisis Service

Donald I. Templer, PhD

Editor's Introduction

Templer's brief chapter makes a harsh point: if Hispanics are denied easy and convenient voluntary access to the mental health care delivery system, their entrance into the system will be coercive.

Previous issues of *Clinical Gerontologist* have dealt with the topics of involuntary commitment:

1991 X (3) 95

and institutionalization:

1985 IV (2) 44-46
1986 IV (3) 41-48
1986 IV (4) 42-45
1986 V 6, 65, 81-84, 86-87, 261, 283, 286-287, 390-392, 493, 507
1986 VI (1) 21-33
1986 VI (2) 13-15, 45-57, 78, 87, 92-93, 101-106, 129-154, 177-188
1987 VII (2) 50-52
1988 VII (3/4) 71-72
1988 VIII (2) 85-88
1989 VIII (4) 24-25
1990 IX (3,4) xi, 1-18

Donald I. Templer is affiliated with California School of Professional Psychology-Fresno.

and reviews of books on that topic

        1982 I (1) 103-104
        1984 III (2) 72-73
        1984 III (1) 86-87
        1987 VII (2) 71-73
        1991 X (3) 95

The entirety of one issue was devoted to how to deal with uncooperative patients.

        1987 VI (2)

The present study was based upon the clinical impression of the author that Mexican-Americans were more likely to be involuntarily brought to the crisis service in an emergency room at a county hospital in California's San Joaquin Valley.

The systematic data collection was over a sixteen month period. An arrival was designated as voluntary if the patient came of his or her own volition and involuntary if the patient was brought by authorities, such as police officers, against his or her will.

Fourteen (35%) of the 40 Mexican-Americans, nineteen (56%) of 34 Blacks, and seventy-five (70%) of 107 Whites had voluntary arrivals ($X^2 = 16.20$, $p < .01$). Thus 35% of Mexican-Americans in contrast to 67% of Blacks and Whites combined ($X^2 = 13.36$, $p < .01$) came voluntarily.

The findings are probably a function to a large extent of persons less assimilated into, and more discriminated against, by the dominant culture being reticent to avail themselves to the services provided by the dominant culture. Also, it is possible that dominant culture health care providers err in considering normal behavior as abnormal because of insufficient knowledge about the subculture. Furthermore, many Mexicans and Mexican-Americans have more faith in their own health practitioners, the Curanderos (Trotter, 1981). Fortunately, there is a growing trend for the rapprochement of Mexican-American and Native American folk healing concepts with dominant culture mental health concepts, both in theory and in practice. It is recommended that this trend be encouraged and promoted. It is also recommended that the families be very much involved from the point of first mental health contact through the implementation of further intervention, maintenance, and prophylactic measures. Needless to say, more Mexican-Americans, both male and female, should be encouraged to go into the mental health professions and should be given adequate support in their education and support.

An example case is that of a 26 year old Mexican-American woman who was brought involuntarily to the emergency room after superficially cutting her wrist. She appeared mildly depressed. She maintained that her actions did not represent serious suicidal intent and that she would not take her life because of her children and her religion. She stated that she was now feeling much better because her family demonstrated much concern regarding the suicidal gesture. The patient said that her husband did not provide her with sufficient consideration. She implied that there may have been more serious marital problems, but she seemed reluctant to discuss such. She was released from the emergency room on the stipulation that she would be seen on an outpatient basis.

A second case is that of a 28 year old Mexican-American man who cut his wrist. He appeared seriously depressed, but his affect also had a flat element. His discourse reflected a looseness of associations, with the content centered primarily upon the magnitude of his depression and his homosexuality and his guilt. He acknowledged auditory hallucinations that included voices commanding him to kill himself. He was admitted to the acute psychiatric unit.

REFERENCE

Trotter, R.T., Chavida, J.A. (1981). *Curanderismo: Mexican-American Folk Healing*. Athens, GA: University of Georgia Press.

Chapter Fourteen

Outreach
to Spanish-Speaking Caregivers
of Persons with Memory Impairments:
A Brief Report

I. Maribel Taussig, PhD
Laura Trejo, MSG, MPA

Editor's Introduction

Taussig and Trejo demonstrate how the mental health care delivery system can use outreach to one group of Hispanic elders: caregivers of dementia patients. A supportive and informative form of workshop is described.

Previous issues of *Clinical Gerontologist* have described community based care:

1990 X (2) 77-79

and approaches to group therapy in general (including group therapy with caregivers):

1982 I (1) 51-58
1983 I (3) 81-90

I. Maribel Taussig is affiliated with the Spanish-Speaking Alzheimer's Disease Research Program, University of Southern California, School of Gerontology. Laura Trejo is affiliated with the Los County Department of Mental Health.

Direct correspondence to: I. Maribel Taussig, PhD, Andrus Gerontology Center, University of Southern California, University Park MC 0191, Los Angeles, CA 90089-0191.

1983 I (4) 19-30
1983 II (2) 23-37
1984 II (3) 25-38
1984 II (4) 37-49
1986 V 231, 239-243, 269, 281-297, 301-307, 385-395, 427
1986 VI (2) 87-88, 141, 143, 147, 149-150
1987 VI (4) 35-60, 70-73
1989 VIII (3) 86-89
1990 IX (3,4) 111-217
1990 X (2) 17-34

as well as reviews of books on group therapy.

1984 II (4) 85-87
1985 III (3) 73-74
1985 IV (2) 82-83
1987 VII (1) 81-82
1988 VII (3/4) 182-183, 189-190
1989 VIII (3) 102-103, 103-104

Organic brain disorders which can result in memory and other cognitive impairments do not appear to discriminate across cultural boundaries, and to some degree, ethnic minority groups may actually experience a higher rate of impairment given past exposure to work related, environmental and other life stresses.

Caregivers of all cultural and racial groups desperately need education and appropriate information to facilitate their caregiving responsibilities. The need is not merely for sharing information but goes further; it is for culturally and linguistically appropriate information to be exchanged at a conferences and workshops.

The purpose of this brief paper is to share the experience of coordinating Spanish-speaking caregivers conferences in Los Angeles County and its degrees of success. The conference topics included: memory impairments, problem solving strategies, identification of community resources and other vital topics associated with meeting the needs of families caring for cognitively impaired older adults.

In May 1989, June and October 1990, conferences were held which reached 175 family caregivers, other family members, advocates, service providers and others who took part in these events. The conferences were made possible through the joint efforts of several agencies/entities committed to providing qualitative information to the Spanish-speaking community.

Alzheimer's disease and other dementing illness are a growing concern of our aging population, and as stated earlier, there is no reason to believe that such illnesses are less common among the Hispanic older population. The number of Hispanics in the USA has increased dramatically in the past 20 years, in California alone, from 1940 to 1980 the numbers have increased from 5.6% to 19.2%. Thus the number of older persons has increased as well. It is well known that the Hispanic older adult is either unable to speak English or if given a choice about 80% prefer to speak Spanish. Much of the available literature regarding Latino caregivers notes the tremendous need for information and the difficulties associated with providing outreach to a monolingual Spanish-speaking community.

An all-day workshop format model (highly utilized by many centers such as Alzheimer's Disease Research Center Consortium of Southern California, and the Saint Barnabas Diagnostic and Treatment Center) was chosen for this conference. The program included lectures and workshops conducted by bilingual professionals working in the field of aging, and a resource fair hosted by local service providers. The program format was composed of three general sessions (myths of aging, an overview regarding dementias, identifying and utilizing community resources). Following the first two general sessions, participants attended a morning and an afternoon workshop selected from four topic-specific areas at registration. These topics included: "Caring for relatives with dementia"; "Legal and financial issues related to caregivers of demented individuals"; "Problem solving"; and "How to talk to your doctor" (see Appendix A for format in Spanish).

Given that this was a day-long workshop, lunch was provided. This unstructured time gave participants the opportunity to interact with one another and with the presenters. Immediately following the afternoon workshops, all participants were assembled again for a general session on community resources. This was followed by a resource fair where local program service providers had an opportunity to answer questions and distribute program literature.

The cost of putting on conferences of this nature requires that adequate income sources be identified. Participants attending these conferences were asked to pay a very small registration fee which included their lunch. Most presenters were paid a small "symbolic" honorarium. Conference coordinators felt most presentors working with these groups are rarely remunerated for their efforts. Yet their expertise is valuable, necessary, and must be treated as such. Money obtained from registrations was not expected to cover all of the costs associated with putting on events of this nature. For this reason, various organizations providing services to the Hispanic community were approached to co-sponsor one or more of the individual conferences.

For most participants, this was their first opportunity to attend a conference of this nature, and they appeared a bit skeptical. Soon we noticed that the degree of questions and their frequency were very similar to those of English-speaking caregivers. During breaks participants began to interact with each other and began to share common problems they were facing. When the conference was over, participants continued interacting with each other, collecting information from the resource fair, and enrolling in various programs.

WHAT HAVE WE LEARNED SO FAR?

These conferences confirmed that the Spanish-speaking community has a great need to learn about dementias, and that their needs are similar to those of non-Hispanic Whites. Participants were especially interested in obtaining information on how to deal with the day-to-day needs of caring for their dementing relatives, what specific services exist, how much they cost, how to qualify for services, and most important, they needed and wanted to share their own knowledge and experiences regarding their own caregiving responsibilities.

We also learned that outreach to this community is not impossible and in fact, most people are willing to attend and participate. That it is most desireable if information such as the flyers are in basic Spanish language without threatening technical words. That if presenters are aware of the culture and social expectations and behaviors of the participants, they will respond in a positive manner, and that if presenters are able to speak the language of the participants they will participate to their fullest.

There are some specific issues which are worth mentioning so that others doing similar projects will not repeat our mistakes. We must first acknowledge that in relation to similar conferences offered to the English-speaking groups, the attendance in numbers were significantly lower. This is most likely because the population targeted is a very specific one, meaning that not only were they Spanish-speaking but also caregivers of demented individuals. We strongly encourage rotation of sites as necessary in order to reach a larger population.

In some areas we could have been more efficient. For example, while the program brochures were developed and disseminated in basic language avoiding technical words, sufficient quantities were not disseminated, nor did we have a "good" mailing list of caregivers addresses for this targeted group.

The centers that were notified regarding this event did not properly communicate to their staff about the event, therefore, many professionals did not convey our message to their clients or patients. The reasons may be many, but, the end result was the same: the caregivers did not hear about the event. Mass media such as radio, television and newspapers were not utilized properly or efficiently. In a city as large as Los Angeles, it is virtually impossible to reach all individuals interested, and when reached, distance makes it virtually impossible for some to attend. In some instances, caregivers wanting to attend did not have someone to care for the impaired person. Therefore, we must be careful not to interpret the small number of individuals participating in this conference as people not wanting or lacking the need for such services.

For all the reasons mentioned above, it is recommended that agencies considering undertaking a project of this nature plan and prepare their program around the following:

Mutual cooperation was one of the key strategies utilized to make this program successful. The co-sponsors of this event were selected because of their interest and deep sense of commitment to the Spanish-speaking community. At the same time, the co-sponsoring agencies/entities all equally shared in the potential success or failure of the program. This strategy was extremely helpful in ensuring that everyone involved worked together towards a successful outcome. It should be noted, that one of the program sponsors was an agency primarily serving an Asian/Pacific Islander population. Their participation served as acknowledgement that the responsibility of developing model programs which serve special target groups can and should be shared across cultural boundaries.

Shared responsibility also carries with it inherent problem areas/needs, such as: the need for identifying and assigning specific tasks, the need for detailed fiscal accountability; the clarification of the various entities mission/goals at the beginning of the planning process, and a clear and documented understanding of what has and has not been agreed to by everyone involved. All of these items play an important role in the successful planning of any event done in conjunction with others.

Patience and trust were also critical factors in the development of this program. For some of the involved co-sponsors this was the first time they worked with other entities. Their ability to take on responsibilities was, at times, dependent on their trust.

Justification for putting on a conference of this type was relatively easy.

In Los Angeles County prior to this event there had not been any program offered for monolingual Spanish-speaking caregivers. Even though, as noted earlier, many programs of this type are offered on an on-going basis by various agencies/entities, none had attempted to fulfill the needs of this target group.

Participant reactions and perceived benefits to the program were many and varied, as were the participants themselves. Those that were shared with program coordinators through verbal comments and program evaluations, include the following:

> The sense of not being alone with these problems.

> The tremendous need for information about memory impairments and available services.

> A shared sense of comfort in knowing that there are professionals trained to meet their needs and who speak their language.

In their aggregate these issues highlight the tremendous and basic need of monolingual communities to have access to the traditional service systems. They also emphasize the neglect by these service systems to be responsive to the needs of an increasingly culturally and linguistically pluralistic society.

Conclusions: The program was successful in the following areas:

1. Reached the target population.
2. Provided needed information.
3. Established the groundwork for future programs.
4. Demonstrated that communities will respond to events which fulfill their needs.
5. Demonstrated to agencies their own capacity to work together to put on a quality program.
6. Taught all of us to keep program attendance, at least for the moment, between 50-70 people to maintain realistic goals.
7. Have a quality environment for participant interaction.

In conclusion we feel that caregivers of all cultural and racial groups need education and appropriate information to facilitate their caregiving responsibilities, and most important that such minorities, in our community, often go without access to needed services because as some put it "They don't come to us," "They take care of their own." Such myths only perpetuate the delay of meaningful and needed programs from reaching already seriously underserved populations.

APPENDIX A

SEGUNDA CONFERENCIA ANUAL PARA LA COMUNIDAD HISPANA

CUIDANDO A NUESTROS SERES QUERIDOS INCAPACITADOS POR PROBLEMAS DE LA MEMORIA

Sábado 6 de Octubre de 1990 • 8:30 a.m. a 3:00 p.m.
Ken Edwards Center, 1527 4th Street, Santa Monica

La meta de esta conferencia es ofrecer información sobre problemas de memoria en las personas mayores y sobre métodos para ayudar a los familiares que tienen a su cargo el cuidado de una persona con estas dificultades. El programa será ofrecido totalmente en español y será conducido por profesionales especializados en asuntos relacionados con personas mayores y su familia.

También participarán representantes de varias agencias los cuales proveerán orientación e información sobre recursos en la comunidad.

La donación para participar es: \$5.00 por persona, esto incluye materiales y almuerzo. Envíe su matrícula antes del 20 de septiembre para reservar su plaza.

Programa/Horario

Maestra de Ceremonias: Livia Bracamonte, M.S.W.

8:30 a.m.	**Matricula/cafe y pan dulce**
9:00 a.m.	**Mitos sobre la vejez** Laura Trejo, M.S.G., M.P.A.
9:30 a.m.	**¡Que es la demencia?** I. Maribel Taussig, Ph.D.
10:15 a.m.	**Descanso**
10:30 a.m.	**Temas variados**

Por favor indique en el formulario de matrícula los dos temas en los que quisiera participar:

A.   **El cuidado de un esposo, padres, o familiares incapacitados**
      Maria P. Aranda, M.S.W., L.C.S.W.

B.   **Asuntos legales y de finanzas relacionados**
      con el cuidado de una persona incapacitada por la demencia
      Robert James Logan, J.D. y Geannie Raya, J.D.

C.   **Cómo convivir eficientemente con**
      el comportamiento de una persona incapacitada por la demencia
      Andres Hernandes. M.S.W., L.C.S.W.

D.   **Cómo utilizar los servicios medicos mas eficientemente**
      Dr. Enrique Montiel

11:45 a.m.	**Almuerzo**
12:45 p.m.	**Temas variados** (Los mismos temas de la mañana serán repetidos)
1:30 p.m.	**¿Qué tipos de servicios existen en la comunidad** **para personas mayores y como utilizarlos?** Rosa Ramirez-Ocasio y Christine Raya-Valencia
2:15 p.m.	**Exhibición de recursos existentes en la comunidad**
3:00 p.m.	**Clausura del programa**

APPENDIXES:
PSYCHOMETRIC SCALES
IN SPANISH TRANSLATION

Appendix I

International Version
of Mental Status Questionnaire

SPANISH TRANSLATION

[This is a test of mental status, not organicity.]

1. ¿Cuántos años tiene usted? (entre dos años)
2. ¿En que año nació¿ (año exacto)
3. ¿En que año estamos¿ (año exacto)
4. ¿En que mes estamos¿ (exacto)
5. ¿Qué comió en su última comida? almuerzo? cena?
6. ¿Cómo se llama este edificio? (nombre o descripción)
7. Cuente los numeros 1 a 10, al reves: 10, 9, 8, et cetera.

[for community elders]

8. ¿Cuál es su dirección?
9. ¿Qué día de la semana es hoy?
10. ¿Quién es el presidente del país?

[for institutionalized elders]

8. ¿Por cuánto tiempo ha estado usted acá en este asilo? (entre 20%)
9. ¿Cómo se llama el director de este asilo?
10. ¿Cómo podríamos llegar al comedor?

Administration & Scoring: Each time that the patient gives an incorrect answer, immediately provide the correct response, telling the patient to try to remember it. After all ten questions have been asked, record the number of initial right answers. Then go back to those questions that the patient missed the first time around and ask them again. Add one point to the patient's *final score* for each repeated item passed. With persons who are immigrants or poorly educated, the final score is a more valid predictor of mental status. The initial score produces too many false positives in these patients. The number of correct answers can be interpreted as follows: 0-3 severe confusion, 4-6 moderate confusion, 7-8 mild confusion, 9-10 lucid and alert.

ANNOTATED BIBLIOGRAPHY ON SPANISH TRANSLATION OF I.V.M.S.Q.

Brink TL: (1979) *Geriatric Psychotherapy*, New York: Human Sciences Press.

Initial presentation of the scale.

Brink TL, Capri D, DeNeeve V, Janakes C & Oliveira, C: (1978) Senile Confusion: Limitations of assessment by mental status questionnaire, face-hand test, and staff ratings. *Journal of the American Geriatrics Society*, 26, 380-382.

The IVMSQ produces false positives for institutionalized elders who are immigrants or poorly educated.

Brink TL, Bryant J, Catalano ML, Janakes C & Oliveira C: (1979) Senile confusion: Assessment with a new stimulus recognition test. *Journal of the American Geriatrics Society*, 27, 126-129.

The IVMSQ correlates .8 with staff ratings, Face-Hand Test and SRT with institutionalized elders.

Brink TL, Janakes C & Martinez L: (1981) Geriatric Hypochondriasis: Situational factors. *Journal of the American Geriatrics Society*, 29, 37-39.

Inter-rater reliability of IVMSQ is .8. Spanish-speaking subjects in the U.S. score significantly lower than English-speaking. Spanish-speaking subjects are more likely to improve significantly on retest.

Brink TL: (1981) Assessment of Senile Confusion in Mexican and Northamerican Aged. Interamerican Psychological Society, Santo Domingo.

Suggests that the Face-Hand Test is the best screening test for avoiding false positives due to cultural factors.

Brink TL, Markoff C, Martinez N, Curran P, Dorr ML, Janson E, McNulty U & Messina M (1986) The Mental Status Questionnaire for

Senile Confusion: Practice effect in English and Spanish Speaking Subjects. *Clinical Gerontologist, 4, #4, 29-35.*

Reviews data from previous studies: Hispanics are more likely to have false positives on dementia tests such as the IVMSQ. Using data from second administration means that the practice effect can be a safeguard against this.

Appendix II

Hypochondriasis Scale
(Institutional Geriatric)

SPANISH TRANSLATION

1. ¿ Está usted generalmente satisfecho con su salud? N
2. ¿ De vez en cuando, se siente usted en salud perfecta? N

   ["Outside of this specific problem . . ." = S]

3. ¿ Se siente usted cansado la mayoría del tiempo? S

   ["I get tired a lot." = N]

4. ¿ Se siente usted mejor en las mañanas? N

   ["Always feel the same." = S]

5. ¿ Tiene usted muchos dolores diferentes? S

   ["I know what they are." = N]

6. ¿ Es deficil creer cuando el médico diga que usted no tiene ningún problema físico? S

   ["He/She knows what's wrong with me" = N]

Administration: These items may be administered in oral or written format, but the former is preferred. The examiner may have to repeat a question in order to get a response that is clearly yes or no.

Scoring: Count one point for each hypochondriacal answer. In both the institutional and community elder populations, the modal score is 0, the median 1. This test is a measure of hypochondriacal attitudes, rather than hypochondriacal behavior. It is possible for a patient to score high (e.g., 4-6) and yet manifest no somatic complaints. Any patient who has numerous somatic complaints and scores high is probably suffering from delusional illness. Any score under 3 is definitely not hypochondriacal, and so the patient's complaints should be taken seriously.

ANNOTATED BIBLIOGRAPHY ON SPANISH
TRANSLATION OF H.S.I.G.

Brink TL, Belanger J, Bryant J, Capri D, Janakes C, Jasculca S & Oliveira C: (1978) Hypochondriasis in an Institutional Geriatric Population: construction of a scale (HSIG). *Journal of the American Geriatrics Society*, 26, 557-559.

Initial presentation of the English version.

Brink TL, Janakes C & Martinez N: (1981) Geriatric Hypochondriasis: situational factors. *Journal of the American Geriatrics Society*, 29, 37-39.

Found inter-rater reliability to be .8, among both English and Spanish speaking community aged. There were no differences between the two groups. There was no correlation with stressful life events.

Brink TL: (1981) Self-ratings of Memory versus Psychometric Ratings of Memory and Hypochondriasis. *Journal of the American Geriatrics Society*, 29, 537-538.

Scores among Mexico City institutionalized aged were comparable to those of American institutionalized aged. Self-ratings of memory did not correlate with objective memory tests, but correlated negatively with the HSIG.

Appendix III

Geriatric Depression Scale

SPANISH TRANSLATION

1. ¿Está usted satisfecho con su vida? N
2. ¿Han dejado de interesarle cosas y actividades que antes lo hacían? S
3. ¿Siente como su vida está vacía? S
4. ¿Se aburre usted con frequencia? S
5. ¿Tiene usted esperanzas en el futuro? N
6. ¿Tiene usted preocupaciones que no se puede quitar de la cabeza? S
7. ¿Está usted de buen humor la mayor parte del tiempo? N
8. ¿Teme que algo malo le suceda? S
9. ¿Se siente contento la mayor parte del tiempo? N
10. ¿A menudo se siente indefenso? S
11. ¿Se siente a menudo nervioso e inquieto? S
12. ¿Prefiere quedarse en casa antes que salir y hacer cosas nuevas? S
13. ¿Se preocupa frecuentemente por el futuro? S
14. ¿Cree que tiene menos memoria que el resto de la gente? S
15. ¿Piensa que es maravilloso estar vivo ahora? N
16. ¿A menudo se siente descorazonado y triste? S
17. ¿Se siente inútil? S
18. ¿Se preocupa por el pasado? S
19. ¿Piensa que la vida es excitante? N
20. ¿Le cuesta empezar nuevos proyectos? S
21. ¿Se siente lleno de energía? N
22. ¿Cree que su situación es desesperante? S
23. ¿Cree que la mayoría de la gente esta mejor que usted? S
24. ¿A menudo se entristece por pequeñas cosas? S
25. ¿Tiene usted a menudo ganas de llorar? S
26. ¿Le cuesta concentrarse? S
27. ¿Se despierta, generalmente, animado? N
28. ¿Evita el contacto social? S
29. ¿Es facil para usted tomar decisiones? N
30. ¿Esta su mente tan clara como siempre? N

[This translation was developed by psychologist Dr. Miguel Angel Gonzalez Felipe, c/o Fernando el Catolico #24, Madrid 280015]

Administration: These items may be administered in oral or written format. If the latter is used, it is important that the answer sheet have printed SI/NO after each question, and the subject is instructed to circle the better response. If administered orally, the examiner may have to repeat the question in order to get a response that is more clearly a yes or no. The GDS loses validity as dementia increases. The GDS seems to work well with other age groups.

Scoring: Count 1 point for each depressive answer. 0-10 = normal; 11-20 = mild depression; 21-30 = moderate or severe depression.

ANNOTATED BIBLIOGRAPHY ON SPANISH TRANSLATION OF G.D.S.

Brink TL, Yesavage JA, Lum O, Heersema P, Adey M & Rose TL: (1982) Screening Tests for Geriatric Depression. *Clinical Gerontologist*, Fall, *1* (#1), 37-43.

Initial English language presentation of GDS.

Brink TL: (1985) Depression in Caribbean Institutionalized Aged: Staff versus test scores. *International Psychologist*, August *27*, (#3), 23-24.

Staff ratings for dementia correlated with tests for dementia, but staff ratings of depression did not correlate with the GDS. Lack of staff training in depressive symptomology was cited as the reason.

Gonzalez F: (1988) Caracteristicas tecnicas y modificaciones introducidas en dos escalas de depresion: estudio piloto para la adaptacion y baremacion de la G.D.S. y el B.D.I. a la poblacion geriatrica espanola. *Psicogeriatria*, *4* (#5), 59-66.

The GDS had higher reliability, and equivalent validity to the BDI within this Spanish sample.

Garcia Pintos C: (1988) Depression and the Will to Meaning: A comparison of the GDS and PIL in an Argentine population. *Clinical Gerontologist*, *7* (3/4), 3-9.

In this sample of Argentine community aged, only 25% scored in the depressed range. Those subjects reporting existential vacuum, or defensiveness, were more likely to be depressed, while those who reported higher levels of meaning, were less likely to be depressed.

Gatewood-Colwell G, Kaczmarek M, Ames MH: (1989) Reliability and Validity of the BDI for a White and Mexican American Population. *Psychological Reports*, *65*, 1163-1166.

GDS correlated .79 with BDI.

Taussig IM: (1989) Translation and Validation of Neuropsychological and Clinical Batteries for Spanish-Speaking Alzheimer's Disease Patients. Presented at International Congress of Gerontology, Acapulco.

Hispanic means and standard deviations on the GDS were comparable to those of Anglos.

Subject Index